Intra Uterine Adhesions

Rahul Manchanda
Editor

Intra Uterine Adhesions

Diagnostic and Therapeutic Insight

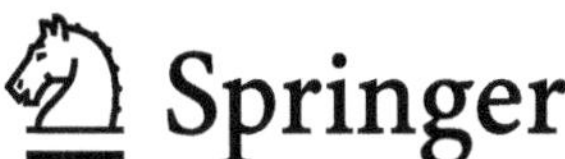

Editor
Rahul Manchanda
Gynae Endoscopy Unit
Pushpawati Singhania Research Institute (PSRI) Hospital
New delhi
Delhi
India

ISBN 978-981-33-4147-0 ISBN 978-981-33-4145-6 (eBook)
https://doi.org/10.1007/978-981-33-4145-6

This Springer imprint is published by the registered company Springer Nature Singapore Pte Ltd.
The registered company address is: 152 Beach Road, #21-01/04 Gateway East, Singapore 189721, Singapore

Foreword

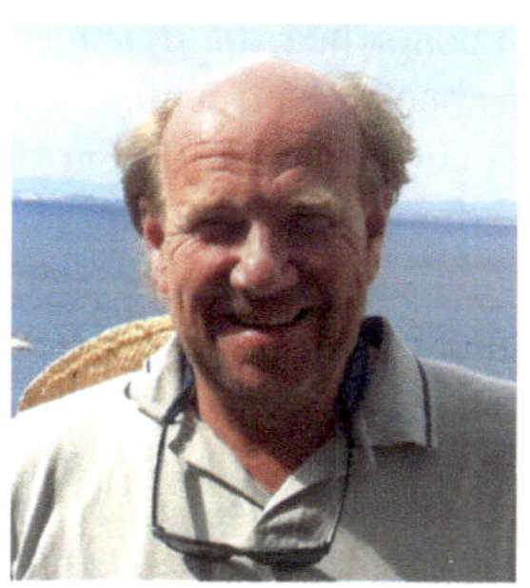

Intrauterine adhesions or synechiae are known since 1894 when they were first described by Heinrich Fritsch (1844–1915). He was a German gynecologist and obstetrician who studied medicine at the Universities of Tübingen, Würzburg, and Halle. From 1893 to 1910, he was a professor at the University of Bonn. Fritsch was a highly regarded surgeon and teacher, who is credited for training an entire generation of acclaimed gynecologists, which included physicians such as Hermann Johannes Pfannenstiel (1862–1909).

In 1927, Bass reported 20 cases of cervical obstruction, in 1500 patients who had undergone induced abortions in a Russian hospital in Rostov. In Copenhagen, in 1946, Stamer described 24 cases of intrauterine adhesions, both postpartum and postabortion associated with intrauterine procedures.

Joseph Asherman (1889–1968), born in Czechoslovakia, received his MD at the University of Prague in 1913. His family emigrated to Israel, and he was working as a gynecologist in Tel Aviv when he described in 1948 (and later in the 50s), frequency, etiology, and symptoms of intrauterine adhesions for the first time in the English language in the Journal of Obstetrics and Gynaecology of The British Empire with the title A*menorrhea traumatica (atretica)*. He defined two entities: traumatic intrauterine adhesions and stenosis of the internal cervical os. Since then, Asherman syndrome has become more common to describe the disease.

Although Asherman's observation was primarily based on a series of cases of intrauterine adhesions occurred after curettage of the gravid uterus, it is now often reported that there are several possible underlying causes of intrauterine adhesions as a result from a traumatic event to the uterine mucosa. This can happen in the gravid and in the nongravid uterus although it is questionable whether the latter variant should be called Asherman syndrome since the pathogenesis in the nongravid uterus is very different from the trauma in the gravid uterus. Trauma to the gravid uterus is the most frequent cause of adhesions; among them are included: miscarriages with curettage, termination of pregnancy with curettage, postpartum curettage, postabortion or postpartum endometritis, ischemic phenomena after postpartum hemorrhage, or uterine artery embolization. For a nongravid uterus, the causes of adhesions include mainly global endometrial ablation, surgical hysteroscopy with resection, or destruction of endometrium on purpose or unintendedly and infections such as genital tuberculosis.

Women with adhesions often struggle with infertility, menstrual irregularities (including amenorrhea, hypomenorrhea, or dysmenorrhea), recurrent pregnancy losses, and a history related to abnormal placentation including praevia and accreta. Hysteroscopy is the method of choice for the diagnosis and treatment of the condition. Various techniques for adhesiolysis and for prevention of scar reformation have been advocated. Surgical success may be defined by the restoration of normal uterine anatomy, by the restoration of normal menses following surgery and by preventing the reformation of intrauterine adhesions.

In this book, all aspects of intrauterine adhesions are covered by various authors, all of which are very well-known specialists in the fields they describe. The reader will find excellent information about the etiology, pathophysiology, clinics, diagnosis, therapy, and prognosis of intrauterine adhesions and Asherman syndrome.

Mark Hans Emanuel
University Medical Center
Utrecht, The Netherlands

University Hospital
Ghent, Belgium

Foreword

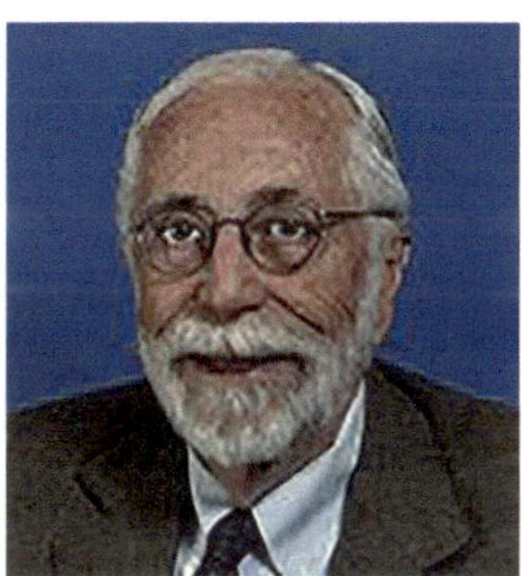

While endoscopy began with Bozzini's work in 1805, it was not until 1869 that Pantaleoni used Desormeaux's endoscope to view the uterine cavity that the first hysteroscopic exam was recorded.

Over the following years, there were problems to be solved before hysteroscopy would become a useful tool for the gynecologist. The resistance of the cervix caused problems of pain which limited its use, and the thick muscle wall of the uterus had to be overcome to create a cavity to view. The latter problem was solved by the introduction of various distending media. But even when these issues were resolved, illumination remained a limiting factor.

Improved optics, cold light sources, and smaller diameter telescopes were valuable advances. However, even with these advances the use of hysteroscopy languished. When I began hysteroscopy in 1973, it was a procedure whose primary indication was to diagnose intrauterine pathology. Some surgical procedures were being considered, but they were not mainstream. Available instrumentation was minimal.

I believe it is fair to say that intrauterine adhesions are the most challenging problem the hysteroscopist faces. The accurate diagnosis of the extent of the problem can be tricky; the surgical expertise required to treat is great, and the prevention of reformation is difficult.

This volume under the editorship of Dr. Rahul Manchanda provides the hysteroscopist with a complete review of this challenging subject. While each chapter could stand alone as an in-depth review of the topic, the logical division of the chapters makes this a valuable reference book.

The strength of the book comes from the authors chosen to write each chapter. Their well-known contributions to the subject allow the reader the opportunity to learn from their experience. Even the expert hysteroscopist will find valuable tips, which can be used in the care of their patients.

Phoenix, AZ Franklin D. Loffer

Foreword

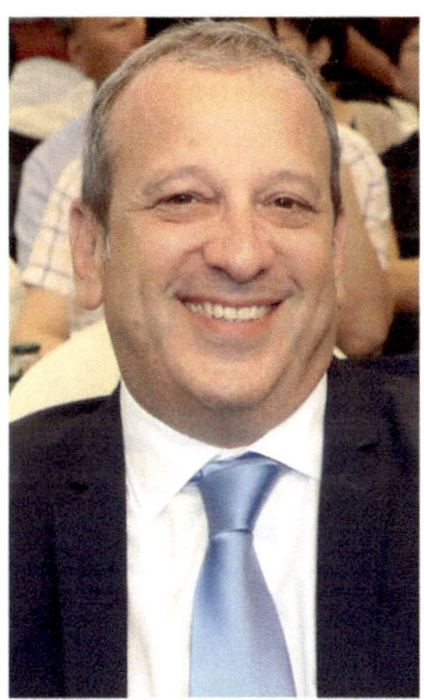

Unfortunately Dilatation and Curettage (D&C) is still one of the most frequent procedures performed on women. D&C is responsible for 90% of all the Asherman syndrome, a syndrome with severe repercussions on the fertility. Hysteroscopic treatment is one of the most difficult and complex procedures, and the perinatal outcome is still poor. These facts help to understand the importance of a book dedicated to such a pathology that I define as "the endometriosis of the hysteroscopy."

This book will help to understand, diagnose, and treat the Asherman syndrome, and also opens a window to the future by showing the innovation related to it.

When Dr. Rahul Manchanda invited me to be part of this project, I felt honored, but when I saw the list of the invited authors names together with the list of chapters, I realized the importance of this book.

Dr. Rahul Manchanda is a talented and enthusiastic professional with a special interest on continues medical education in gynecology endoscopy with an emphasis on hysteroscopy, passion that we share.

This book will mark a before and an after on what we know on Asherman syndrome and is very recommended.

S. Haimovich
Del Mar University Hospital
Barcelona, Spain

Hillel Yaffe Medical
Center/Technion—Israel Technology Institute
Hadera, Israel

Preface

Sadly the topic "intrauterine adhesions" is missing in most books. A subject considered too humble to justify the time or space. Thus ignorance has led to this neglect. Yet they have the ability to prevent the normal physiology and rhythm of the uterus and disrupt its and even prevent its valuable functions.

Ashermans is but a small part of this vast subject but best known as it has had the most attention in diagnosis and treatment.

Here a worldwide group of leading hysteroscopic surgeons have given of their time, knowledge, and experience and also generously shared their expertise to bring this subject to light.

This book discusses all aspects of this pathology from its history, epidemiology, and pathogenesis to the diagnosis, management, and follow-up.

It is one of the first of its kind if not the first that addresses this condition in all aspects while looking at the present evidence available.

Hysteroscopy is the gold standard for diagnosis and management and that is where this book emanates from.

The authors in the chapters, who are renowned in their field and are from different parts of the world, take you through the journey from history to the newer concepts and techniques to management of complications.

It is a book, which is for all family health-care providers, gynecologists, and obstetricians, infertility specialists, endoscopic surgeons, and hysteroscopists.

New Delhi, India — Rahul Manchanda

Acknowledgments

This book has probably been long time coming, longer than even I have known. It started with the experience that one got from tackling this pathology during one's practice.

Hence I must first thank my teachers and patients who have been the foundation of this treatise.

I thank Springer and its team for making this book a reality.

I thank all the chapter authors from all over the world who have contributed generously of their knowledge and experience.

Mr. Bhuvan Mishra, I owe you a thank you for all your help.

My family, Mum, Bhavna, Anya, and Anvi, I am fortunate to have you all, thank you.

Contents

1 **History and Epidemiology** 1
Péter Török

2 **Etiopathogenesis of Asherman's Syndrome** 7
Jose Carugno, Douglas Timmons, and Michael Saad Naguib

3 **Clinical Features (Signs and Symptoms)** 13
Miguel Angel Bigozzi, Laura Amoresano, and Jorge E. Dotto

4 **Intrauterine Adhesions: Classification Systems** 21
Rahul Manchanda and Aayushi Rathore

5 **Diagnosis: Patient Evaluation (Flowchart)** 33
Antonio Simone Laganà, Simone Garzon, Gaetano Riemma, and Salvatore Giovanni Vitale

6 **Ultrasound Diagnosis and Management** 41
Ashok Khurana

7 **Role of Hysterosalpingography (HSG) and Sono-HSG** 61
Nitin P. Ghonge, Sanchita Dube Ghonge, and Alka Ashmita Singhal

8 **Diagnostic Hysteroscopy** 89
Sergio Haimovich

9 **Overview and Treatment: Hysteroscopic Techniques** 103
Ferdinando Murgia, Fabiana Divina Fascilla, and Stefano Bettocchi

10 **Role of Assisted Operative Hysteroscopy in Asherman's Management** 123
Jude E. Okohue

11 **Postoperative Care (Hormonal Therapy, Physical Barriers, Vasodilators, Antibiotics)** 137
Sarah Gustapane, Bruno Francesco Barba, and Andrea Tinelli

12 Organic Tissue Grafts Following Intrauterine Adhesiolysis 149
Mohammed Amer and Mounir Mostafa

13 Follow-Up and Relook Hysteroscopy 163
Attilio Di Spiezio Sardo, Maria Chiara De Angelis, Antonella D'Apolito, Jose Carugno, and Gloria Calagna

14 Complications and Fertility Potential Following Adhesiolysis 173
Luis Alonso Pacheco, Jose Carugno, Douglas Timmons, and Marta Garcia Sanchez

15 Pregnancy and Its Management: Post-Asherman's Treatment 185
Kamal Buckshee and Tanya Buckshee Rohatgi

16 Placental Complications Associated with Asherman's Syndrome 199
Salvatore Giovanni Vitale, Federica Di Guardo, and Antonio Simone Laganà

About the Editor

Rahul Manchanda, MD, FICOG, FICMCH, FICS, FACS is the Director of Manchanda's Endoscopic Center, New Delhi, and Head of the Gynae Endoscopy Unit at Pushpawati Singhania Research Institute (PSRI) Hospital, New Delhi. His areas of interest are safe hysteroscopy, Asherman's syndrome, and hysteroscopy in adenomyosis. He has many publications in international and national journals and is a reviewer with many international journals. He has organized and is an active operative faculty in various international and national conferences.

Dr. Manchanda is a renowned faculty master in endoscopy and minimally invasive gynecological surgery, Bologna University, Italy, Founder cochairperson of International Hysteroscopy Congress, and the Indian representative on the scientific committee of Global Hysteroscopy Congress and Newsletter.

He is a FOGSI (Federation of Obstetricians and Gynecologists of India), ICOG (Indian College of Obstetricians and Gynecologists), and IAGE (Indian Association of Gynecological Endoscopy) accredited endoscopy teacher.

1 History and Epidemiology

Péter Török

IUAs usually occur as a result of trauma to the basal layer of the endometrium. IUAs with symptoms of hypomenorrhea or amenorrhea, infertility, and recurrent pregnancy loss are referred to as Asherman's syndrome [1]. For cases without symptoms asymptomatic intrauterine adhesion designation should be used.

The bands of fibrous tissue that are formed in the endometrial cavity in response to uterine procedures are called intrauterine adhesions (IUAs). The original description of Asherman's syndrome was based on intrauterine adhesions produced after curettage of the gravid uterus, but there are several other possible underlying causes (intrauterine operative procedures) of intrauterine adhesions.

1.1 History

Asherman's was first described in 1894 by Heinrich Fritsch, as a case of posttraumatic intrauterine adhesion. Several authors published intrauterine adhesions as single cases: Austrian gynecologist Ernst Wertheim (1864–1920), Otto Ernst Küstner (1849–1931), Gustav von Veit (1824–1903), and Josef Halban (1870–1937).

In 1927 Bass reported 20 cases of cervical obstruction in a series of 1500 patients who had undergone induced abortions.

Stamer reviewed 37 cases reported in the literature in 1946 and added 24 cases of his own with intrauterine adhesions associated with gravid uterus.

Joseph G. Asherman (1889–1968) published his work first in 1948 to describe the frequency, etiology, symptoms, and roentgenologic picture of this condition.

P. Török (✉)
Faculty of Medicine, Department of Obstetrics and Gynecology, University of Debrecen, Debrecen, Hungary

R. Manchanda (ed.), *Intra Uterine Adhesions*,
https://doi.org/10.1007/978-981-33-4145-6_1

1.1.1 Synonymous Are

- Fritsch syndrome
- Intrauterine adhesions (IUAs)
- Intrauterine synechiae
- Endometrial sclerosis
- Traumatic uterine atrophy
- Fritsch-Asherman syndrome [2]

1.2 Epidemiology

It is impossible to detect or estimate the true prevalence of all IUAs, as probably most cases are without symptoms. Only cases with AS, which imply pain, bleeding disorders, or impaired fertility, need treatment.

The prevalence ranges from 1.5% to 45.5% as an incidental finding. Reasons of this wide range can be the difference among the evaluated population, intrauterine operative procedure, instrument, and diagnostic method that was used.

Increasing prevalence of IUAs could be the result of more intrauterine procedures, but it can also be increased due to more effective diagnostic methods. Ultrasound with better resolution and the more widespread use of ambulatory office-hysteroscopy can be the reasons for cases being recognized more [3].

A predisposition to intrauterine adhesions could be linked to unspecific factors like age, race, geographical area, and nutritional status. In Denmark, a total of 61 unique cases of AS were found during a 10-year period, in Holland 638 women with AS were referred to a specialist center during a 10-year period, and in Saudi Arabia, 41 women were referred with AS to a specialist center during an 8-year period [4]. Chen et al. found 357 cases of AS in a 4-year period in a large women's hospital in China [5].

Any kind of intrauterine procedures can cause adhesions in the uterine cavity as a postoperative complication. Due to the status of the uterus (gravid or nongravid) outcomes could be different.

After reviewing 1856 cases, Schenker and Margalioth [6] found pregnancy as a disposing factor in 90.8%.

In the background, low level of estrogen can play a role that is needed for the regeneration of the endometrium. After pregnancy (delivery, miscarriage, or abortion) basal layer of the endometrium could be in vulnerable state, so it is more sensitive for the mechanical lesions. The basal layer appears to be most susceptible to damage in the first 4 weeks following delivery or abortion.

The development of IUA can occur after Cesarean section, postabortion/miscarriage curettage, postpartum curettage, cesarean section, and evacuation of a hydatidiform mole.

IUA's prevalence was found to be 15% or 19% after spontaneous abortion followed by D&C.

Repeated curettage following pregnancy loss also increases the risk of developing adhesions. Odds of IUA are almost double for patients with more than one miscarriage, compared to those with one.

Intrauterine gynecological procedures can cause IUAs, as well. In Schenker's [6] study Asherman's syndrome was diagnosed in 1.6% (30 out of 1856) after diagnostic curettage, and 1.3% (24 out of 1856) following abdominal myomectomy. Taskin et al. [7] found that the frequency of Asherman's syndrome was 6.7% (1 out of 15) of patients after resection of uterine septa. There are more data in literature, where IUA formation was detected after some more infrequent interventions, e.g., after bilateral uterine artery embolization (UAE) and uterine devascularization because of severe postpartum hemorrhage or any types of endometrial ablations (thermal balloon ablation 36.4%, and other types).

According to some authors, inflammatory processes do contribute to the damaging effect of trauma and act synergistically in the formation of IUAs. In a prospective cohort study, 35% of cases with known IUAs had confirmed chronic endometritis [8].

Schenker's [6] study reported genital tuberculosis as a causing factor in 4% (74 cases).

1.2.1 Pathology

The extent of the endometrial damage may not directly correlate with the severity of the symptoms. For obstructive amenorrhea, the lesion is often focal and limited to the uterine isthmus and cervical canal. A biopsy of the fundal part of the uterine cavity often reveals normal or inactive endometrium.

Histologically, Asherman's syndrome is a condition in which the endometrium becomes fibrosed. The endometrial stroma is largely replaced by fibrous tissue, and the glands are usually represented by an inactive cubo-columnar epithelium of the endometrial type. The distinction between the functional and basal layer of the endometrium is lost; the functional layer is replaced by an epithelial monolayer, which is nonresponsive to hormone stimulation; and fibrous synechiae form across the cavity. In other cases, there may be calcification or even ossification in the stroma, and the glands may be sparse and inactive or cystically dilated. Vascularity might be abundant, containing thin-walled dilated vessels, but in most cases the tissue becomes avascular.

Adhesions may involve different layers of the endometrium, myometrium, or connective tissue. Adhesions derived from each of these tissues exhibit a characteristic hysteroscopic picture. Endometrial adhesions are quite similar in appearance compared with the surrounding endometrium. Myofibrous adhesions, which are most often encountered, are characterized by the presence of a thin layer of overlying endometrium, the surface of which is furnished with many glandular ostia. The surface of connective tissue adhesions lacks an endometrial lining and contrasts markedly with the adjacent endometrium. Fibrous adhesions that show dense connective tissue exhibit no lining in contrast to surrounding endometrium.

1.2.2 Some Minutes

- The prevalence of AS in women with impaired fertility ranges from 2.8% to 45.5% depending on the subpopulation [9] and the prevalence of AS to be 4.6% among an infertile population [10].
- It is found in 1.5% of women evaluated with a hysterosalpingogram (HSG) for infertility, between 5% and 39% of women with recurrent miscarriage.
- The incidence of IUA varies between 15% and 40% after curettage [11]. After secondary removal of placental remnants or repeat curettage after incomplete abortion a prevalence of IUA was 40% [12].
- Prevalence of IUA was 19.1% diagnosed by hysteroscopy within 1 year in women diagnosed with miscarriage treated expectantly, medically, or surgically [13].
- Incidence of IUA was 10% after one curettage evaluated by HSG and after two curettages the incidence was 30.6%, when evaluated by hysteroscopy at 10 weeks after the curettages [14, 15].
- Significantly more IUAs are found after curettage compared to hysteroscopic removal (35.9% vs. 4.2%) among women with retained products of conception (RPOC) after delivery or miscarriage [16].
- First-trimester procedures cause less severe adhesions, the majority with grades 1–2 (ESGE classification) compared to postpartum procedures, where the majority have grades 3–5 [1].
- Asherman's syndrome may occur in 31% of women after the initial hysteroscopic resection of leiomyoma, and up to 46% after the second hysteroscopic resection.

Key Points
1. Heinrich Fritsch, as a case of posttraumatic intrauterine adhesion, first described Asherman's in 1894.
2. Joseph G. Asherman (1889–1968) published his work first in 1948 to describe the frequency, etiology, symptoms, and roentgenologic picture of this condition.
3. The prevalence can range from 1.5% to 45.5% as an incidental finding.
4. Any kind of intrauterine procedures can cause adhesions in the uterine cavity as a postoperative complication.
5. The extent of the endometrial damage may not directly correlate with the severity of the symptoms.

References

1. Hanstede MMF, van der Meij E, Goedemans L, Emanuel MH. Results of centralized Asherman surgery, 2003–2013. Fertil Steril. 2015;104:1561–8.
2. Yu D, Wong YM, Cheong Y, Xia E, Li TC. Asherman syndrome—one century later. Fertil Steril. 2008;89(4):759–79.
3. Lagana AS, Ciancimino L, Mancuso A, Chiofalo B, Rizzo P, Triolo O. 3D sonohysterography vs. hysteroscopy: a cross-sectional study for the evaluation of endouterine diseases. Arch Gynecol Obstet. 2014;290(6):1173–8.

4. Kjer JJ. Asherman syndrome in a Danish population. Acta Obstet Gynecol Scand. 2014;93(4):425–7.
5. Chen L, Zhang H, Wang Q, et al. Reproductive outcomes in patients with intrauterine adhesions following hysteroscopic adhesiolysis: experience from the largest women's hospital in China. J Minim Invasive Gynecol. 2017;24(2):299–304.
6. Schenker JG, Margalioth EJ. Intrauterine adhesions: an updated appraisal. Fertil Steril. 1982;37:593–610.
7. Taskin O, Sadik S, Onoglu A, Gokdeniz R, Erturan E, Burak F, Wheeler JM. Role of endometrial suppression on the frequency of intrauterine adhesions after resectoscopic surgery. J Am Assoc Gynecol Laparosc. 2000;7:351–4.
8. Chen Y, Liu L, Luo Y, et al. Prevalence and impact of chronic endometritis in patients with intrauterine adhesions: a prospective cohort study. J Minim Invasive Gynecol. 2017;24:74.
9. March CM, Israel R, March AD. Hysteroscopic management of intrauterine adhesions. Am J Obstet Gynecol. 1978;130(6):653–7.
10. Baradwan S, Baradwan A, Al-Jaroudi D. The association between menstrual cycle pattern and hysteroscopic March classification with endometrial thickness among infertile women with Asherman syndrome. Medicine. 2018;97(27):e11314.
11. Salzani A, Yela DA, Gabiatti JRE, Bedone AJ, Monteiro IMU. Prevalence of uterine synechia after abortion evacuation curettage. Sao Paulo Med J. 2007;125(5):261–4.
12. Westendorp IC, Ankum WM, Mol BW, Vonk J. Prevalence of Asherman's syndrome after secondary removal of placental remnants or a repeat curettage for incomplete abortion. Hum Reprod. 1998;13(12):3347–50.
13. Hooker AB, Lemmers M, Thurkow AL, et al. Systematic review and meta-analysis of intrauterine adhesions after miscarriage: prevalence, risk factors and long-term reproductive outcome. Hum Reprod Update. 2014;20:262–78.
14. Tsapanos VS, Stathopoulou LP, Papathanassopoulou VS, Tzingounis VA. The role of Seprafilm bioresorbable membrane in the prevention and therapy of endometrial synechiae. J Biomed Mater Res. 2002;63(1):10–4.
15. Hooker AB, de Leeuw R, van de Ven PM, et al. Prevalence of intrauterine adhesions after the application of hyaluronic acid gel after dilatation and curettage in women with at least one previous curettage: short-term outcomes of a multicenter, prospective randomized controlled trial. Fertil Steril. 2017;107(5):1223–31.
16. Rein DT, Schmidt T, Hess AP, Volkmer A, Schöndorf T, Breidenbach M. Hysteroscopic management of residual trophoblastic tissue is superior to ultrasound-guided curettage. J Minim Invasive Gynecol. 2011;18(6):774–8.

2 Etiopathogenesis of Asherman's Syndrome

Jose Carugno, Douglas Timmons, and Michael Saad Naguib

Intrauterine adhesions are bands of fibrous tissue that occur inside the endometrial cavity frequently in response to endometrial injury. The severity of this condition can range from thin strings of filmy tissue to complete obliteration of the cavity with subsequent amenorrhea and infertility among other clinical devastating consequences. Clinical challenges include primary prevention of adhesions and prevention of recurrent adhesions after surgical treatment. In this chapter, we provide an overview of the etiopathogenesis of intrauterine adhesions.

2.1 Etiology

The most common cause of Asherman's syndrome is trauma to the endometrium. This can be the result of a dilation and curettage (D&C) for spontaneous abortion or termination of pregnancy, a molar pregnancy, or a curettage in the postpartum period (Fig. 2.1). Due to this knowledge, the rate of medical abortions to avoid surgical manipulation has risen in some parts of the world [1]. In a study of 1856 cases examined by Schenker and Margalioth, pregnancy was the predominant risk factor, and 66.7% of Asherman's cases occurred after postabortion/miscarriage curettage, 21.5% after postpartum curettage, 2% after cesarean section [2], and 0.6% after evacuation of hydatidiform mole [3]. Rare cases of IUAs have been seen in C-sections even after the use of B-lynch procedure in the event of postpartum hemorrhage.

It remains unknown why pregnancy has a high risk of Asherman's. One of the theories is that the low estrogen status of the patient before and after the procedure does not allow for adequate growth and stimulation of the endometrium [4].

J. Carugno (✉) · D. Timmons · M. S. Naguib
Obstetrics, Gynecology and Reproductive Sciences Department, Minimally Invasive Gynecology Unit, University of Miami, Miller School of Medicine, Miami, FL, USA

R. Manchanda (ed.), *Intra Uterine Adhesions*,
https://doi.org/10.1007/978-981-33-4145-6_2

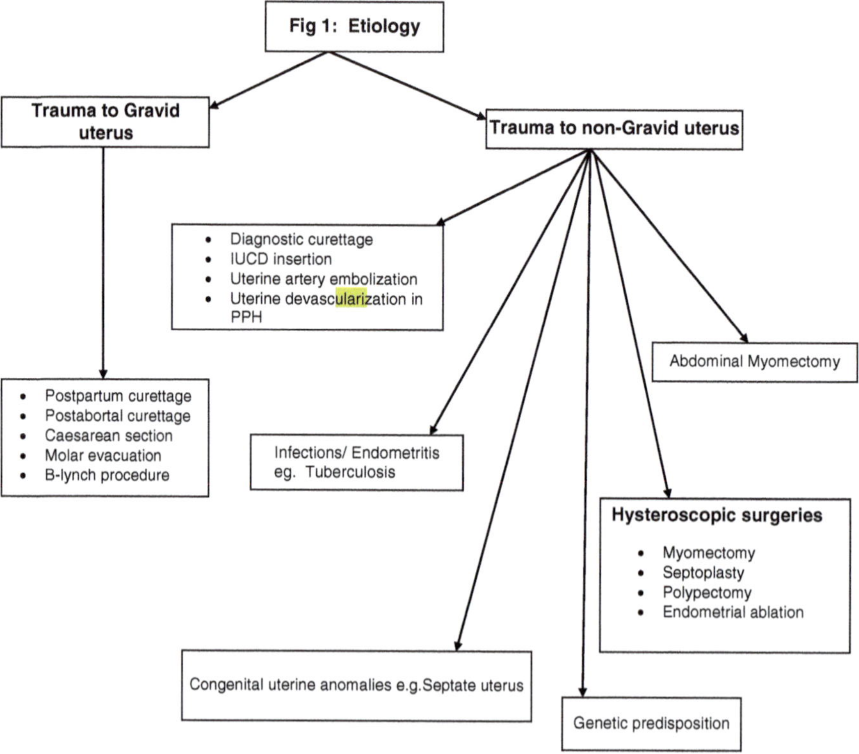

Fig. 2.1 Etiology

Another possible reason for the higher risk brought by pregnancy is that the uterus may be in a more vulnerable state after pregnancy, thus causing the basal layer of the endometrium to be more easily damaged by trauma [4]. This is supported by the observation that a large percentage of patients with Asherman's report prior instrumentation after pregnancy. Studies show that the risk of adhesion development is higher when the procedure is performed in the 2nd to 4th postpartum weeks (21.5–40%), and the risk is actually lower if endometrial manipulation is performed within 48 h [2]. One of the theories of increased adhesion formation in postabortion D&Cs is that the placental remnants can encourage fibroblastic activity and collagen formation, causing adhesions before the endometrium can regenerate [3].

Other causes of Asherman's syndrome are manipulation of the uterus or endometrium. As reported by Yu et al., Asherman's syndrome was seen after diagnostic curettage (1.3%), hysteroscopic resection of uterine septum (6.7%), hysteroscopic myomectomy (31–45%), abdominal myomectomy, insertion of IUD (0.2%), and even uterine artery embolization [1] (Table 2.1).

Asherman's can also occur after endometrial ablation (36.4%). This is logical as the ablation destroys the basal layer of the endometrium in order to prevent

Table 2.1 Relation between risk factors and frequency of occurrence of Asherman's

Risk factors	Frequency [6] (%)
Miscarriage curettage	66.7
Postpartum curettage	21.5
Caesarean section	2
Trophoblastic disease evacuation	0.6
Mullerian duct malformation	16
Infection (genital tuberculosis)	4
Diagnostic curettage	1.6
Abdominal myomectomy	1.3
Uterine artery embolization	14
Hysteroscopic surgery: metroplasty	6
Insertion of IUCD	0.2
Uterine compressive sutures for PPH	18.5
Hysteroscopic surgeries	
Metroplasty	6
Myomectomy (single myoma)	31.3
Myomectomy (multiple myomas)	45.5
Endometrial ablation	36.4
Polypectomy	0.3
Septoplasty	6.7

the regrowth of endometrium. Unlike in the above cases where patients may desire future fertility, the majority of individuals undergoing endometrial ablation do not wish to maintain childbearing ability. The rate of IUAs after ablation may be even higher as these patients will not come with a complaint of a decrease in menstrual flow as decreased menses is an expected effect of endometrial ablation.

Infection has also been proposed as a cause of Asherman's syndrome. The method by which infection can cause this is still hotly debated. In a report of 171 patients who underwent cesarean section, 28 developed endometritis; however, postoperative hysterosalpingogram (HSG) demonstrated no difference in intrauterine adhesions between the endometritis group and the rest of the group [4].

Despite being a rare etiology in the United States, genital tuberculosis has been identified as a more common and concerning cause of IUAs in developing countries such as India. In these patients, the uterine cavity is totally obliterated, and the endometrium is destroyed. These patients go on to experience amenorrhea and infertility [4]. The damage caused by genital TB is so severe that attempts to repair the endometrial cavity are often futile [2].

Along with the above causes, another possible cause or risk factor for Asherman's is congenital anomalies of the uterus, specifically a septate uterus [4]. No studies have been done to determine whether the anomaly was the cause of Asherman's. It is thought that the uterine anomaly places the patient at risk for multiple hysteroscopic procedures, thus placing the patient at higher risk of developing adhesions [4]. Lastly, reports of Asherman's syndrome after pelvic radiation have also been reported [5].

2.2 Pathogenesis

After trauma or the abovementioned causes of Asherman's occur, the basal layer of the endometrium is damaged and becomes fibrosed, and the stroma is exchanged for fibrous tissue [5]. Unfortunately, the molecular mechanisms regulating the pathogenesis of adhesions are not known at this time [4].

Changes at the cellular level occur, with the endometrium transforming to an inactive cubo-columnar epithelial layer [4]. The distinction between the basal layer and the functional layer becomes nonexistent, and there is no longer a differentiation between the functional and basal layer of the endometrium as the functional layer is replaced by an inactive avascular layer in which fibrous synechiae form across the cavity. The fibrotic synechiae disrupt the entire cavity, and on relook hysteroscopy, stromal calcifications and ossification are seen [2]. The new fibrous layer of tissue is not responsive to hormone stimulation [4]. The fibrous adhesions exhibit dense connective tissue and demonstrate no endometrial lining in comparison to the surrounding endometrium (Fig. 2.2).

At the histological level, when full-thickness myometrial biopsies were taken, it was found that the uterine wall was 50–80% fibrous tissue in comparison to 13–20% of control subjects [4]. In addition, Asherman's has also been noted with deep adenomyosis [1]. With such a large amount of the endometrium being replaced by

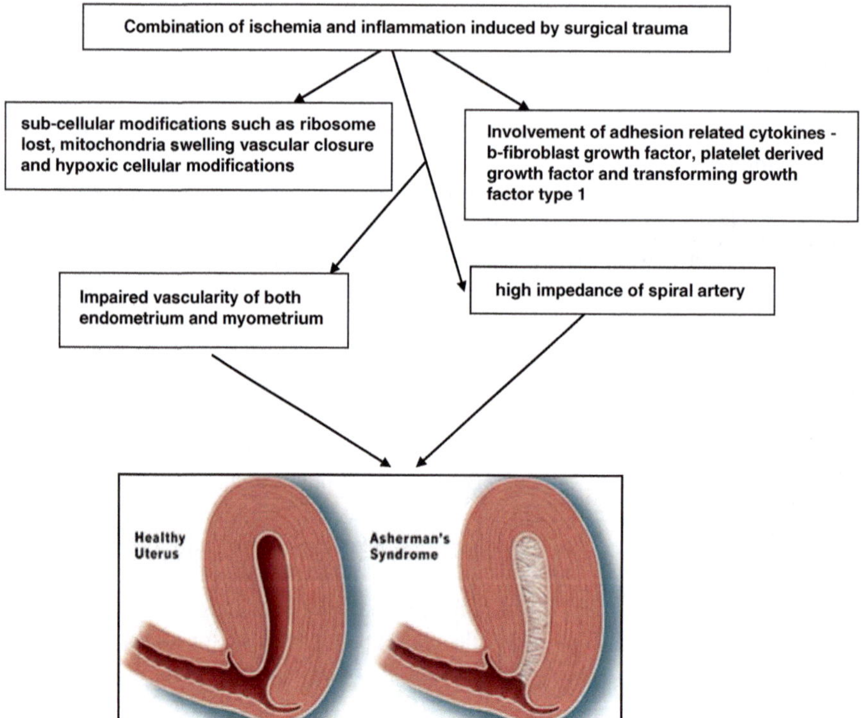

Fig. 2.2 Pathogenesis

fibrous adhesions, it is thought that the myometrial activity is thus decreased, and the perfusion of hormones is inhibited as well.

Common cytokines known to be involved in the pathogenesis of adhesions include TGF-β, TNF-α, IL-1, and IL-18 [7]. Their exact role is yet to be determined. In a study by Wang et al., it was noted that NF-kB was significantly elevated in the endometrium of patients with Asherman's. NF-kB is a transcription factor that promotes the expression of IUA inflammatory markers and is seen as a major component of inflammatory disease [7]. More studies are planned by this group to further determine the possible clinical role of NF-kB.

Other possible causes for the pathogenesis of adhesions include the cytokine b-fibroblast growth factor, platelet-derived growth factor, and transforming growth factor type 1 [6]. Further work must be done to confirm their role in Asherman's as well.

Lastly, it has been hypothesized that there is a genetic component in the formation of IUAs; however, there is scant evidence on what genetic factors may be involved [6]. Moving forward, several studies will be performed so that a better understanding of Asherman's is obtained, which may help physicians with treatment and prevention of this devastating pathology.

Key Points

1. Intrauterine adhesions are bands of fibrous tissue that occur inside the endometrial cavity frequently in response to endometrial injury.
2. The most common cause of Asherman's syndrome is trauma to the endometrium.
3. Main pathophysiology includes combination of ischemia and inflammation induced by surgical trauma.
4. Genital tuberculosis has been identified as a more common and concerning cause of IUAs in developing countries such as India.
5. Miscarriage curettage accounts for 66.7% and postpartum curettage accounts for 21.5% risk of AS.

References

1. Dreisler E, Kjer JJ. Asherman's syndrome: current perspectives on diagnosis and management. Int J Women's Health. 2019;11:191–8.
2. Malhotra N, Bahadur A, Kalaivani M, Mittal S. Changes in endometrial receptivity in women with Asherman's syndrome undergoing hysteroscopic adhesiolysis. Arch Gynecol Obstet. 2012;286(2):525–30.
3. Schenker JG. Etiology of and therapeutic approach to synechia uteri. Eur J Obstet Gynecol Reprod Biol. 1996;65(1):109–13.
4. Yu D, Wong YM, Cheong Y, Xia E, Li TC. Asherman syndrome—one century later. Fertil Steril. 2008;89(4):759–79.
5. Salazar CA, Isaacson K, Morris S. A comprehensive review of Asherman's syndrome: causes, symptoms and treatment options. Curr Opin Obstet Gynecol. 2017;29(4):249–56.
6. Conforti A, Alviggi C, Mollo A, De Placido G, Magos A. The management of Asherman syndrome: a review of literature. Reprod Biol Endocrinol. 2013;11:118.
7. Wang X, Ma N, Sun Q, Huang C, Liu Y, Luo X. Elevated NF-kappaB signaling in Asherman syndrome patients and animal models. Oncotarget. 2017;8(9):15399–406.

3 Clinical Features (Signs and Symptoms)

Miguel Angel Bigozzi, Laura Amoresano, and Jorge E. Dotto

Intrauterine adhesions cause total or partial obliteration of the endocervix and/or uterine cavity, resulting in hypomenorrhea or amenorrhea, infertility, and pregnancy loss. The majority of patients with IUAs present with menstrual abnormalities, usually hypomenorrhea or secondary amenorrhea. Others may have relatively normal menses and in which case a high index of suspicion is needed to make diagnosis.

Endometrium is composed of two layers, the functional layer (adjacent to the uterine cavity) which is shed during menstruation, and an underlying basal layer (adjacent to the myometrium), which is necessary for regenerating the functional layer.

Trauma to the basal layer, typically after a dilation and curettage (D&C) performed after a miscarriage, or delivery, or for surgical termination of pregnancy, can lead to the development of intrauterine scars resulting in adhesions that can obliterate the cavity to varying degrees. In extreme cases, the whole cavity may be scarred and occluded. Even with relatively few scars, the endometrium may fail to respond to estrogen.

Dan Yu et al. proposed the following criteria for the diagnosis of Asherman's syndrome [1]:

M. A. Bigozzi (✉)
Head of Hysteroscopy Unit, Hospital B. Rivadavia, Buenos Aires, Argentina

Board ISGE, Argentine Medical Society of Hysteroscopy, Buenos Aires, Argentina

L. Amoresano
Head of Hysteroscopy Unit, Hospital B. Rivadavia, Buenos Aires, Argentina

J. E. Dotto
Board ISGE, Argentine Medical Society of Hysteroscopy, Buenos Aires, Argentina

Department of Gynecology, Buenos Aires University, Buenos Aires, Argentina
e-mail: jdotto@intramed.net.ar

R. Manchanda (ed.), *Intra Uterine Adhesions*,
https://doi.org/10.1007/978-981-33-4145-6_3

1. One or more clinical features: amenorrhea, hypomenorrhea, subfertility, recurrent pregnancy loss, or a history related to abnormal placentation including previa and accreta
2. The presence of intrauterine adhesions by hysteroscopy and/or histologically confirmed intrauterine fibrosis

3.1 Clinicopathological Association

The clinical features are closely associated with pathologic findings like depth of fibrosis, location of adhesions, and extent of pathologic changes.

The location of the adhesion can include the cervical canal, uterine cavity, or both cervical canal and uterine cavity.

Obstructive amenorrhea is a consequence of intracervical adhesions or stenosis, and patients often present with amenorrhea with periodic abdominal discomfort. There may be a normal uterine cavity and thus a good prognosis after treatment. The most common variety is when the adhesions are in the uterine cavity.

3.1.1 Subcategories

- *Central intrauterine adhesion without constriction of the cavity*: Patients with central intrauterine adhesions always have some normal endometrium and a relatively normal cavity. Therefore, the prognosis after treatment is usually good.
- *Partial obliteration of the cavity with constriction*: Patients with partial obliteration of the cavity have a reduced and irregular cavity.
- *Complete obliteration of the cavity*: No cavity is found and it results in amenorrhea.

In all of these conditions, the patient may present with any symptoms and the extent of disease can be confirmed by hysteroscopy. The extent will influence the prognosis.

The prognosis for pregnancy in these patients is often poor.

In some cases, the adhesions can be located in both cervical canal and cavity of the uterus. The patient may present with any symptoms, including menstrual abnormalities, infertility, and pregnancy complications, and the outcome (such as normal menses and fertility) depends very much on the severity and extent of the adhesions.

3.2 WHRIA's (Women's Health & Research Institute of Australia) Stages of Asherman's Syndrome

3.2.1 Stage I

- Minor scarring in either the cervical canal or the uterine cavity.
- Unless this involves isthmus, there will be little impact on the normal function of the uterus and treatment is not essential.

- If the scar involves the isthmus, there can be a significant impact on the function of the endometrium.
- Most women are able to conceive.

3.2.2 Stage II

- Patients frequently present at this stage of the condition.
- There will be an obstruction of the internal os.
- In some women this obstruction involves only a fraction of a millimeter; in others it can stretch over several centimeters.
- If the scarring involves the isthmus, there will be no menses and pain, or there will be mild cramps with no bleeding.
- Women with stage II Asherman's syndrome have more than a 60% chance of conceiving again.

3.2.3 Stage III

- The uterus will normally contract and more than 50% is blocked by scar tissue.
- There may also be an obstruction of one of the tubal orifices.
- The greater the extent of scar formation, the more difficult it is to treat.
- Typically, women have less than a 30% chance of successfully conceiving and delivering a child.

3.2.4 Stage IV

- More than 75% of the uterus is blocked and it is smaller in size.
- Treatment at this stage requires multiple visits and has a low success rate.
- Stem cell technology may improve the outcome.

3.3 Spectrum of Clinical Features

3.3.1 Gynecological Features (Fig. 3.1)

3.3.1.1 Menstrual Disorders

Menstrual disorders appear in 48–75% [2] of the patients with intrauterine adhesions. It is characterized by a decrease in flow and duration of bleeding (amenorrhea, scanty bleeding, or infrequent bleeding). Menstrual abnormalities are not always related to the severity of the disease.

- ***Hypomenorrhea*** may be caused by the replacement of normal endometrium by fibrosis, as well as endometrial trauma where damaged endometrium does not

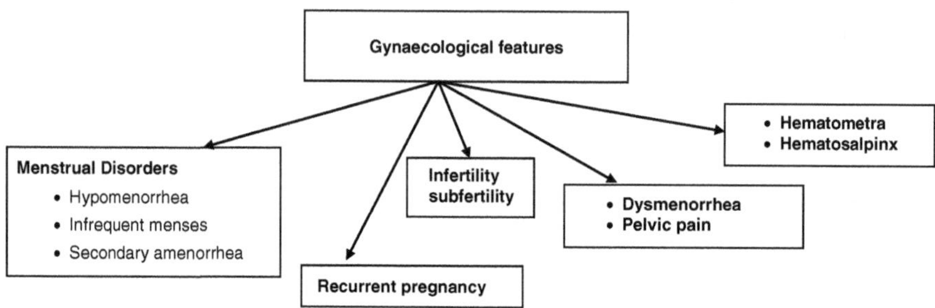

Fig. 3.1 Gynecological features

respond to estrogenic stimulus, as it would under normal conditions. The vascular damage to the tissues may precede the development of Asherman's syndrome.

- ***Amenorrhea***
  1. Cervical adhesions blocking menstrual flow.
  2. Severe endometrial fibrosis leading to destruction of the entire basal layer of the endometrium.
- ***Dysmenorrhea*** is occasionally present (3.5%).
- ***Atretic amenorrhea***: Mechanical obstruction of the internal cervical os could lead to secondary amenorrhea, periodic discomfort or pain, hematometra [3], and even hematosalpinx.

3.3.1.2 Infertility

Infertility appears in about 50% of patients diagnosed with Asherman's syndrome [3]. It may occur when the endometrium fails to respond to hormonal stimulation, as well as a restricted endometrial area [3].

Infertility could be due to occlusion of the tubal ostia, uterine cavity, or cervical canal caused by adhesions, which could prevent the migration of sperm or implantation of the embryo.

3.3.1.3 Recurrent Pregnancy Loss

The World Health Organization (WHO) defines recurrent pregnancy loss as two clinical pregnancy losses, not necessarily consecutive. Intrauterine adhesions and endometrial damage result in a restricted endometrial area and lead to abnormal placentation associated to recurrent pregnancy loss [4]. Some studies report early pregnancy loss (up to 13 completed weeks of pregnancy) in 25–40% [5] of these patients.

3.3.1.4 Causes for Recurrent Pregnancy Loss

1. Constriction of the uterine cavity caused by adhesions
2. Insufficient amount of normal endometrial tissue to support implantation and development of the placenta
3. Inadequate vascularization of the residual endometrial tissue due to fibrosis

3.4 Obstetrical Problems (Fig. 3.2)

Upon achieving pregnancy, obstetrical complications are more frequent.

Schenker and Margalioth [6] reported that among 165 pregnancies in women with untreated Asherman's syndrome, the rate of spontaneous miscarriage was 40% (66 out of 165), preterm delivery was 23% (38 out of 165), term delivery was 30% (50 out of 165), placenta accreta was 13% (21 out of 165), and ectopic pregnancy was 12% (2 out of 165).

The defective placentation may lead to fetal growth restriction (FGR). There have been several cases of FGR described in pregnant women with Asherman's syndrome after endometrial ablations. The defective uterine endometrium and obliterated uterine cavity may also predispose women to ectopic tubal and cervical pregnancies.

3.4.1 Fetal Growth Restriction (FGR) and Low Birth Weight

Endometrial trauma and restricted placental and uterine blood flow result in fetal growth restriction and low-birth-weight babies.

A retrospective research [7] conducted on 56 women, 14 cases, and 42 examinations concluded that pregnant patients diagnosed with Asherman's syndrome gave birth to children weighing less (2.23 ± 0.28 kg) than healthy pregnant women (3.13 ± 0.383 kg).

3.4.2 Abnormal Placentation

Endometrial damage leads to abnormal placentation, increasing the risk of placenta previa, ectopic pregnancy, and placenta accreta [8]. Placenta accreta would be caused by basal layer of the endometrial trauma leading to an increased invasion of the trophoblasts. Schenker and Margalioth [6] found an incidence of placenta

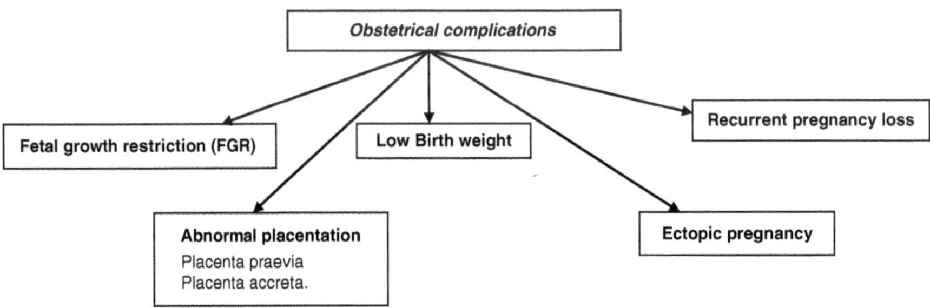

Fig. 3.2 Obstetrical complications

accreta in 13–14% of patients with previous Asherman's syndrome. Roy et al. [9] reported an incidence of postpartum hemorrhage due to adherent placenta in 12.5% of the women who had undergone hysteroscopic adhesiolysis due to Asherman's syndrome.

Any patient with a previous history of intrauterine surgery or Asherman's syndrome should be thoroughly examined by a skilled sonographer for possible abnormal placentation. In case of any suspicion of abnormal placentation, the patient should be scheduled for planned cesarean section with a setup of skilled clinicians due to risk of severe postpartum hemorrhage.

3.4.3 Ectopic Pregnancy

Asherman's syndrome, preceding uterine curettage, previous delivery by cesarean section, and cervix or uterine surgery are considered as underlying risk factors of ectopic pregnancy [10]. These conditions are associated to tissue damage leading to an abnormal placentation. The obliteration of the uterine cavity is also an underlying cause of tubal and cervical ectopic pregnancy.

3.4.4 Differential Diagnosis

Symptoms of the following disorders can be similar to Asherman's syndrome. Comparisons may be useful for a differential diagnosis:

- ***Primary amenorrhea***: Failure of menstruation by the age of 15 years or failure of breast development and menses by 13 years of age. Most often this disorder is a result of immaturity of hypothalamo-pituitary-gonadotropin axis. Symptoms of primary amenorrhea may be the absence of secondary sex characteristics, incomplete or underdeveloped external genitalia and breasts, ovarian deficiency, underactive pituitary, and an absence of menstruation. Secondary amenorrhea occurs in Asherman's syndrome, following D&C or acute endometritis.
- ***Endometriosis***
- ***Pelvic Inflammatory Disease (PID)***
- ***Stein-Leventhal Syndrome***

Key Points

1. Asherman's syndrome results in hypomenorrhea, amenorrhea, and infertility.
2. Patients with Asherman's syndrome may experience pelvic pain and/or hematometra.
3. Obstetrical complications are more frequent among patients with Asherman's syndrome.
4. Endometrial trauma may result in fetal growth restriction, low birth weight, and abnormal placentation.

References

1. Yu D, Wong YM, Cheong Y, Xia E, Li TC. Asherman syndrome—one century later. Fertil Steril. 2008;89(4):759–79.
2. Takai IU, Kwayabura AS, Ugwa EA, Idrissa A, Obed JY, Bukar M. A 10-year review of the clinical presentation and treatment outcome of Asherman's syndrome at a center with limited resources. Sci Res. 2015;5(6):442–6.
3. Panayotidis C, Weyers S, Bosteels J, et al. Intrauterine adhesions (IUA): has there been progress in understanding and treatment over the last 20 years? Gynecol Surg. 2009;6:197.
4. Ford HB, Schust DJ. Recurrent pregnancy loss: etiology, diagnosis, and therapy. Rev Obstet Gynecol. 2009;2(2):76–83.
5. Valle RF. Intrauterine adhesions (Asherman's syndrome). In: Office and operative hysteroscopy. France: Springer-Verlag; 2002. p. 230–2.
6. Joseph G, Schenker MD, Ehud J, Margalioth MD. Intrauterine adhesions: an updated appraisal. Am Fert Soc. 1982;37(5):596–606.
7. Baradwan S, Baradwan A, Bashir M, Al-Jaroudi D. The birth weight in pregnant women with Asherman syndrome compared to normal intrauterine cavity: a case-control study. Medicine (Baltimore). 2018;97(32):e11797.
8. Engelbrechtsen L, Langhoff-Roos J, Kjer JJ, Istre O. Placenta accreta: adherent placenta due to Asherman syndrome. Clin Case Rep. 2015;3(3):175–8.
9. Roy KK, Baruah J, Sharma JB, Kumar S, Kachawa G, Singh N. Reproductive outcome following hysteroscopic adhesiolysis in patients with infertility due to Asherman's syndrome. Arch Gynecol Obstet. 2010;281:355–61.
10. Verma U, Maggiorotto F. Conservative management of second-trimester cervical ectopic pregnancy with placenta percreta. Fertil Steril. 2006;87(3):697. e13–6

Intrauterine Adhesions: Classification Systems

4

Rahul Manchanda and Aayushi Rathore

4.1 Background

Intrauterine adhesions (IUA) were first reported by Heinrich Fritsch in the late nineteenth century. However, its etiology, symptoms, and diagnosis were later described in detail by Joseph Asherman in 1948 [1].

The term intrauterine adhesion is often used interchangeably with Asherman syndrome. But having said that, there is still a very subtle difference between the two terms. IUA refers to the fibrotic bands that form between the walls of the uterus as a result of trauma to the endometrium. Asherman syndrome incorporates the complete spectrum of disease, which includes the formation of intrauterine adhesions resulting in the clinical manifestations like menstrual dysfunction with or without cyclical abdominal pain, infertility, and poor reproductive outcomes.

It has long been known that endometrial injury (especially of the gravid uterus) is the leading cause of Asherman syndrome. It causes damage to the basal layer of the endometrium, which gets subsequently replaced with fibrous tissue. This is the key event in the development of intrauterine adhesions and associated symptoms [2]. The main risk factors causing this injury include curettage of pregnant uterus, mullerian anomaly, infections, uterine surgeries, and compressive sutures for postpartum hemorrhage [1].

Previously, HSG was widely used for the diagnosis of Asherman syndrome. The role of ultrasound, saline infusion sonography, and MRI has also been evaluated.

R. Manchanda (✉)
HOD, Gynaecology Endoscopy Unit, PSRI Hospital, New Delhi, India

A. Rathore
VMMC & Safdarjang Hospital, New Delhi, India

R. Manchanda (ed.), *Intra Uterine Adhesions*,
https://doi.org/10.1007/978-981-33-4145-6_4

However, with the advent of hysteroscopy, it has become the gold standard and the investigation of choice for the diagnosis of Asherman syndrome.

Classification of Asherman syndrome according to its severity was necessary, to ensure better prognostication of patients and for better postoperative follow-up and for assessing the adequacy of treatment.

4.2 HSG-Based Classification

Initial attempts to classify Asherman syndrome were based on the individual HSG findings. It started in 1978 with **Toaff and Ballas** conducting a study to determine the impact of the extent of adhesions as well as their location in the uterus on the menstrual pattern of patients by using HSG [3]. Their findings were classified as follows:

- **Grade 1**: a single, small, filling defect, well inside the uterine cavity, occupying up to about one-tenth of the uterine area (Fig. 4.1)
- **Grade 2:** a single, medium-sized filling defect occupying one-fifth of the uterine area, or several smaller defects adding up to the same degree of involvement, located inside the uterine cavity, whose outline may show minor indentations but no gross deformation (Fig. 4.2)
- **Grade 3**: a single, large or several smaller, filling defects involving up to about one-third of the uterine cavity, which is deformed or asymmetrical because of marginal adhesions (Fig. 4.3)
- **Grade 4**: large-sized filling defects occupying most of the severely deformed uterine cavity (Fig. 4.4)

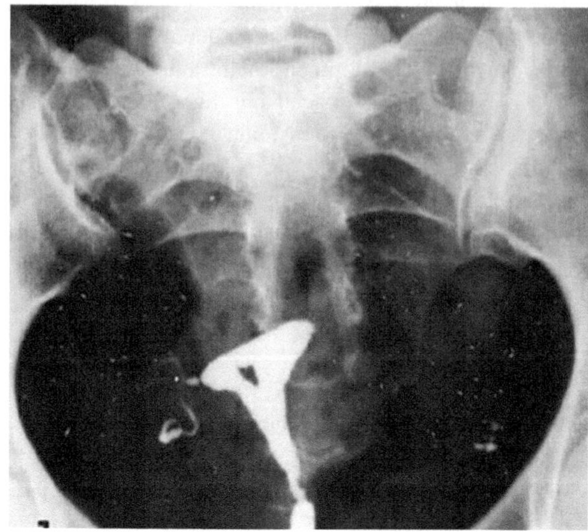

Fig. 4.1 Grade 1 corporeal adhesions

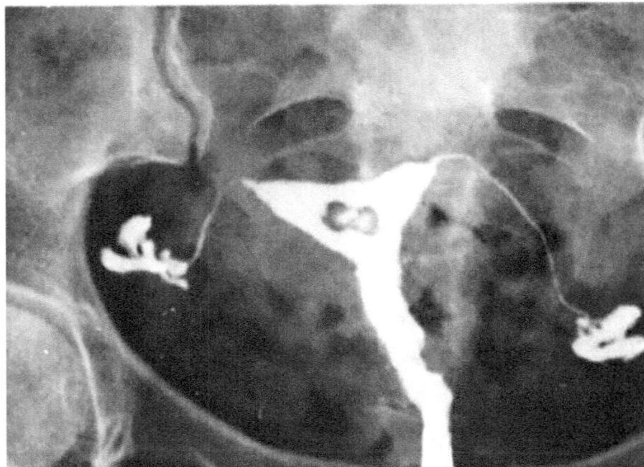

Fig. 4.2 Grade 2 corporeal adhesions

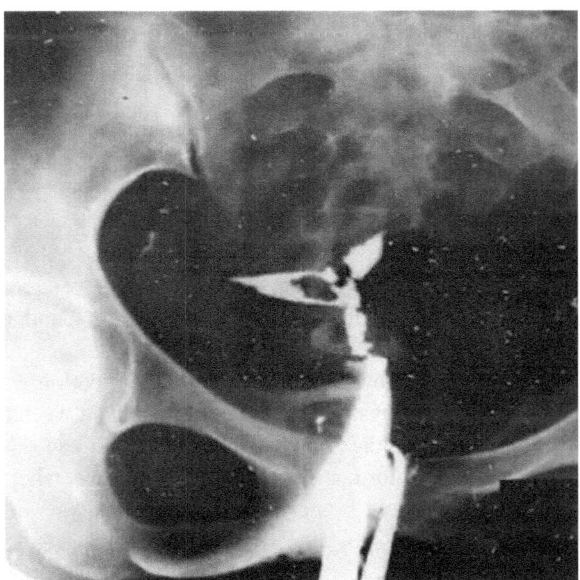

Fig. 4.3 Grade 3 corporeal adhesions

Later, with the increasing use of hysteroscopy, by virtue of its advantages over HSG, it was anticipated to be a better classification tool. Over the subsequent years, all efforts were focused to build an ideal hysteroscopy-based classification system.

4.3 Hysteroscopy-Based Classification

In 1978, **March** became the pioneer in developing a hysteroscopy-based classification system [4]. His aim was to grade the severity of Asherman syndrome according to the extent of coverage of endometrial cavity by adhesions and the degree of occlusion of the uterine cavity. According to this classification system, Asherman

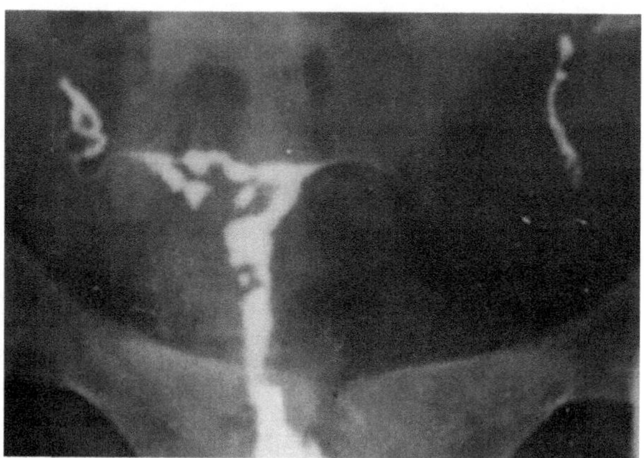

Fig. 4.4 Grade 4 corporeal adhesions

Table 4.1 Classification of Asherman syndrome by March 1978

Classification	Involvement
Severe	>3/4th uterine cavity involved, agglutination of walls or thick bands, ostial areas and upper cavity occluded
Moderate	1/4th to 3/4th uterine cavity involved, no agglutination of walls, adhesions only, ostial areas and upper fundus only partially occluded
Minimal	<1/4th uterine cavity involved, thin or flimsy adhesions, ostial areas and upper fundus minimally involved or clear

syndrome can be of minimal, moderate, and severe category. The simplicity of its use makes it a popular classification used in clinical settings even to this day (Table 4.1).

He argued that hysteroscopy-based classification was better for standardization of individual findings, for ease of comparison between the different dissection techniques, and that choice and extent of treatment can be decided on the basis of this classification. He further advocated that in severe Asherman syndrome, second-look hysteroscopy should be performed, as adhesiolysis in such cases can be difficult at once.

The drawback of his study was that he made no attempt to correlate this severity of the disease with the degree of success of treatment.

In 1983 **Hamou et al**. declared that only identifying the degree of uterine cavity involvement was not sufficient for classification of Asherman syndrome and that the size and histologic nature of adhesions as well as the assessment of the surrounding glandular endometrium were equally important and should be included in the classification system [5] (Table 4.2).

In his study he used a micro-hysteroscope with 4 mm diameter and 30-degree fore-oblique lens with CO_2 distension media for hysteroscopic adhesiolysis. At first the endometrial cavity was examined under panoramic view to determine the extent of intrauterine adhesions. This was then followed by contact hysteroscopy for assessment of size and histologic nature of adhesions under 20× magnification. The thickness, extension, and glandular nature of the surrounding endometrium were later inspected under 60× and 150× magnification (after methylene blue staining).

Table 4.2 Classification of Asherman syndrome by Hamou, 1983

Location of adhesions	Isthmic
	Marginal
	Central
Size of adhesions	<1 cm^2
	>1 cm^2
Type of adhesions	Endometrial adhesions
	Fibrous/connective tissue adhesions
	Myometrial adhesions

Table 4.3 Classification of Asherman syndrome by Valle, 1988

Type of adhesion	Mild
	Moderate
	Severe
Extent of uterine cavity occlusion	Partial
	Total

It was upheld that hysteroscopy-based classification system was more useful than HSG-based classification, in planning treatment and guiding further follow-up.

He identified three different varieties of adhesions in his study:

- *Endometrial adhesions*: white, vascularization similar to surrounding endometrium
- *Fibrous or connective tissue adhesions*: transparent, bridge-like, and poorly vascularized
- *Myometrial adhesions*: highly vascular and extensive adhesions

In 1988, **Valle** likewise devised another hysteroscopy-based classification system including the extent of uterine cavity involvement as well as the type of adhesions [6]. In addition to this, for the first time he suggested that success of treatment (identified by improvement in menstrual pattern and reproductive outcomes) should also be correlated with the severity of disease.

The different types of adhesions were defined as follows:

- *Mild:* flimsy adhesions, composed of endometrial tissue producing partial or complete uterine cavity occlusion
- *Moderate*: fibromuscular adhesions, composed of endometrium causing partial or total occlusion of the uterine cavity, can bleed on adhesiolysis
- *Severe*: dense connective tissue adhesions, lacks endometrial tissue and causes partial or total occlusion of the uterine cavity, not likely to bleed on adhesiolysis

He reported that the best results were obtained in case of mild adhesions and partial occlusion of uterine cavity and less satisfactory results were achieved with severe adhesions and complete occlusion of the cavity (Table 4.3).

Table 4.4 Classification of Asherman syndrome by Donnez and Nisolle, 1994

Degree	Location
I	Central adhesion
	(a) Thin flimsy adhesion (endometrial adhesions)
	(b) Myofibrous (connective adhesions)
II	Marginal adhesions (always myofibrous or connective)
	(a) Wedge-like projection
	(b) Obliteration of one horn
III	Uterine cavity absent on HSG
	(a) Occlusion of the internal os (upper cavity normal)
	(b) Extensive coaptation of the uterine walls (absence of the uterine cavity, true Asherman syndrome)

In 1994, Donnez and Nisolle proposed yet another classification system which reinstated the role of HSG along with hysteroscopy in the classification system. He broadly divided Asherman syndrome into three groups and six subgroups depending on the type of adhesion and the extent of uterine involvement [7] (Table 4.4).

4.4 Clinico-Hysteroscopic Classification

Prior to this time, the classification systems formulated were subjective which chiefly relied on the diagnostic modality used, i.e., HSG or hysteroscopy. None of these included the clinical symptoms of the patient in categorizing the severity of the disease.

In 1988, the American Fertility Society (AFS) provided a comprehensive classification system for Asherman syndrome which has become the most widely accepted classification system over the years [8]. It was the first to include clinical symptom (menstrual pattern) as a part of the categorization. Assessment of menstrual function of the patient was important as it gave a clue to how much of the endometrium was available for post-adhesiolysis regeneration.

Scoring points (1–3) were assigned to each of the included characteristics and staging of Asherman was done as stage 1/2/3 (mild/moderate/severe) according to the score obtained. Additionally, prognostic scoring can be carried out for each patient using this system. Hence, this was a more objective way of classification (Table 4.5, Fig. 4.5).

The European Society of Hysteroscopy (ESH) further designed a classification system including the menstrual pattern in 1989 [9]. However, reproductive outcome of patients was once again not included as a separate entity in this classification. It is a more complex grading system in which Asherman syndrome was categorized under six groups as tabulated below. As it is more cumbersome to use, it did not gain as much popularity as the AFS classification (Table 4.6).

More recently, **Nasr** (in 2000) gave the clinico-hysteroscopic scoring system [10]. It is the most exhaustive and so far an ideal classification system because it includes the clinical symptoms (both menstrual pattern and reproductive outcome)

Table 4.5 Classification of Asherman syndrome by the American Fertility Society, 1988

	Characteristics		
Extent of cavity involved	<1/3	<1/3–2/3	>2/3
	1	2	4
Type of adhesions	Flimsy	Flimsy and dense	Dense
	1	2	4
Menstrual pattern	Normal	Hypomenorrhea	Amenorrhea
	0	2	4
Prognostic classification		HSG score	Hysteroscopy score
Stage I (mild)	1–4		
Stage II (moderate)	5–8		
Stage III (severe)	9–12		

Patient's Name ______ Date ______ Chart # ______
Age ____ G ____ P ____ Sp Ab ____ VTP ____ Ectopic ____ Infertile Yes ____ No ____
Other Significant History (i.e. surgery, infection, etc.) ______

HSG ______ Sonography ______ Photography ______ Laparoscopy ______ Laparotomy ______

Extent of Cavity Involved	<1/3	1/3 - 2/3	>2/3
	1	2	4
Type of Adhesions	Filmy	Filmy & Dense	Dense
	1	2	4
Menstrual Pattern	Normal	Hypomenorrhea	Amenorrhea
	0	2	4

Prognostic Classification		HSG* Score	Hysteroscopy Score
Stage I (Mild)	1-4	______	______
Stage II (Moderate)	5-8	______	______
Stage III (Severe)	9-12	______	______

*All adhesions should be considered dense

Treatment (Surgical Procedures): ______

Prognosis for Conception & Subsequent Viable Infant*
______ Excellent (> 75%)
______ Good (50-75%)
______ Fair (25%-50%)
______ Poor (< 25%)

*Physician's judgment based upon tubal patency.

Recommended Followup Treatment: ______

Property of
The American Fertility Society

Additional Findings: ______

DRAWING

HSG Findings

Hysteroscopy Findings

For additional supply write to:
The American Fertility Society
2140 11th Avenue, South
Suite 200
Birmingham, Alabama 35205

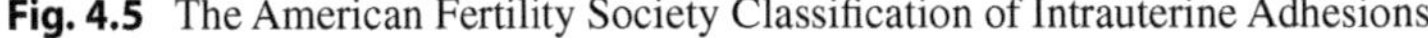

Fig. 4.5 The American Fertility Society Classification of Intrauterine Adhesions

of the patient and the hysteroscopy findings and also gives a prognostic correlation (Table 4.7).

In this new system of classification, greater emphasis is given to the type of adhesions and the ability to visualize the tubal ostia over the involvement of rest of the cavity.

The types of adhesions were classified as flimsy/dense/tubular cavity. Here tubular cavity signifies the most severe form of the disease, which indicates dense adhesions obliterating the entire uterine cavity, thereby obscuring both the tubal ostia.

Table 4.6 Classification of Asherman syndrome by the European Society of Hysteroscopy, 1989

Grade	Extent of intrauterine adhesion
I	Thin or flimsy adhesion
	Easily ruptured by hysteroscope sheath alone
	Corneal areas normal
II	Singular firm adhesions
	Connecting separate parts of the uterine cavity
	Visualization of both tubal ostia possible
	Cannot be ruptured by hysteroscope sheath alone
IIa	Occluding adhesions only in the region of internal cervical os
	Upper uterine cavity normal
III	Multiple firm adhesions
	Connecting separate parts of the uterine cavity
	Unilateral obliteration of ostial areas of tubes
IIIa	Extensive scarring of the uterine cavity wall with amenorrhea or hypomenorrhea
IIIb	Combination of III and IIIa
IV	Extensive firm adhesion with agglutination of uterine walls
	At least both tubal ostial areas occluded

Table 4.7 Classification of Asherman syndrome by Nasr, 2000

Hysteroscopic findings		Score
Isthmic fibrosis		2
Flimsy adhesions	Few	1
	Excessive (>50% of the cavity)	2
Dense adhesions	Single band	2
	Multiple bands (>50% of the cavity)	4
Tubal ostium	Both visualized	0
	Only one visualized	2
	Both not visualized	4
Tubular cavity (sound <6)		10
Menstrual pattern		
Normal		0
Hypomenorrhea		4
Amenorrhea		8
Reproductive performance		
Good obstetric history		0
Recurrent pregnancy loss		2
Infertility		4

0–4 = mild (good prognosis)
5–10 = moderate (fair prognosis)
11–12 = severe (poor prognosis)

In addition to this, isthmic fibrosis has been included as a separate entity as it can initiate a neuroendocrine reflex and can cause amenorrhea even when the rest of the cavity is free of adhesions.

4.5 Recent Updates

In India, recently in 2016, another hysteroscopy-based classification system was introduced which is known as the **MEC (Manchanda's Endoscopic Center) classification of Asherman syndrome** (Table 4.8). It also categorized Asherman syndrome as mild, moderate, and severe disease owing to the extent of involvement of the uterine cavity. It incorporates both dense and flimsy adhesions in all the categories. The core advantage of using this system is that it is a relatively simple classification and can be easily applied in the clinical settings while performing hysteroscopy. It makes the planning of treatment and follow-up of patients even more convenient [11].

A retrospective study done in 2018 by Sharma et al. based on the MEC classification correlated the reproductive outcome of women with the severity of the disease and reported an increased number of live birth rates in moderate and severe category of adhesions. In this study the direction and degree of hysteroscopic adhesiolysis were guided by the preoperative assessment of myometrial thickness of fundal, anterior, and posterior walls using the "RR" method [12].

4.5.1 Guidelines for Classification of Intrauterine Adhesions

AAGL in collaboration with ESGE, in 2017, formulated the following guidelines on intrauterine adhesions:

1. Intrauterine adhesions should be classified, as prognosis is correlated with severity of adhesions: Level B.
2. The various classification systems make comparison between studies difficult to interpret. This may reflect inherent deficiencies in each of the classification systems. Consequently, it is currently not possible to endorse any specific system: Level C [13].

Table 4.8 MEC classification of Asherman syndrome

Grade	Category	Characteristics
Grade 1	Mild	Less than 1/3rd of uterine cavity obliterated (flimsy/dense adhesions)
Grade 2	Moderate	1/3rd to 2/3rd of uterine cavity obliterated (flimsy/dense adhesions)
Grade 3	Severe	More than 2/3rd of uterine cavity obliterated (flimsy/dense adhesions)

4.6 Conclusion

Changes in the menstrual pattern of a woman or poor reproductive outcomes in a woman with a history of endometrial trauma point to the diagnosis of Asherman syndrome. In all suspected cases, attempt should be made to classify the disease according to its severity and treatment plan should be formulated accordingly. An ideal classification system should include comprehensive analysis of the disease symptoms along with the extent of uterine involvement. Additionally, prognostic scoring should be done and further follow-ups should be scheduled along those lines.

Gradually over a period of time, a variety of classification systems were proposed, each having its own benefits and disadvantages. Having said that, none of the classifications specify the impact of severity of Asherman syndrome on the reproductive outcome of the patient. Moreover, these systems have not yet been validated through clinical studies and hence further research must be done to predict the clinical application of these classification systems. The summary of various classification systems used is shown in Table 4.9.

Table 4.9 Classification systems for Asherman syndrome/IUA

Source	Summary of classification
Toaff and Ballas	Classification into 4 grades to determine the impact of the extent of adhesions as well as their location in the uterus on the menstrual pattern of patients by using HSG
March et al.	Adhesions classified as minimal, moderate, or sever based on hysteroscopic assessment of the degree of uterine cavity involvement
Hamou et al.	Adhesions classified as isthmic, marginal, central, or severe according to hysteroscopic assessment
Valle and Sciarra	Adhesions classified as mild, moderate, or severe according to hysteroscopic assessment and extent of occlusion (partial or total) at HSG
European Society for Hysteroscopy	Complex system classifies IUAs as grades I through IV with several subtypes and incorporates a combination of hysteroscopic and HSG findings and clinical symptoms
American Fertility Society	Complex scoring system of mild, moderate, and severe IUAs based on the extent of endometrial cavity obliteration, appearance of adhesions, and patient menstrual characteristics based on hysteroscopy or HSG assessment
Donnez and Nisolle	Adhesions classified into 6 grades on the basis of location, with postoperative pregnancy rate the primary driver. Hysteroscopy or HSG is used for assessment
Nasr et al.	Complex system creates a prognostic score by incorporating menstrual and obstetric history with IUA findings at hysteroscopic assessment
Chitra et al.	A simple and easy-to-use classification system dividing Asherman into 3 grades: mild, moderate, and severe according to the extent of uterine involvement on hysteroscopy (MEC classification)

Key Points

1. Classification of Asherman syndrome is necessary to evaluate the extent of intrauterine adhesions, selecting the best treatment option and analyzing the postoperative success of adhesiolysis.
2. The various classification systems include HSG-based classification, hysteroscopy-based classification, and clinico-hysteroscopic classification.
3. Currently HSG-based classifications have become obsolete and there has been a shift towards using hysteroscopy-based classification.
4. The most widely accepted among these is the AFS classification which is a clinico-hysteroscopic classification.
5. On the other hand, the most comprehensive classification system was developed by Nasr in 2000 which is the most ideal one, to include prognostic scoring as well as the reproductive outcome of the patients.
6. The most recent classification system has been developed in 2016 in India, known as MEC classification, which is hysteroscopy based and is relatively simple and easy to implement under clinical settings.
7. Further clinical studies are required to validate the clinical application of these classification systems and to prognosticate the patients about their posttreatment reproductive outcomes according to the severity of the condition.

References

1. Conforti A, Alviggi C, Mollo A, De Placido G, Magos A. The management of Asherman syndrome: a review of literature. Reprod Biol Endocrinol. 2013;11:118. https://doi.org/10.1186/1477-7827-11-118.
2. Amin TN, Saridogan E, Jurkovic D. Ultrasound and intrauterine adhesions: a novel structured approach to diagnosis and management. Ultrasound Obstet Gynecol. 2015;46(2):131–9. https://doi.org/10.1002/uog.14927.
3. Toaff R, Ballas S. Traumatic hypomenorrhea-amenorrhea (Asherman syndrome). Fertil Steril. 1978;30(4):379–87. https://doi.org/10.1016/s0015-0282(16)43568-5.
4. March CM, Israel R, March AD. Hysteroscopic management of intrauterine adhesions. Am J Obstet Gynecol. 1978;130:653–7.
5. Hamou J, Salat-Baroux J, Siegler AM. Diagnosis and treatment of intrauterine adhesions by microhysteroscopy. Fertil Steril. 1983;39:321–6.
6. Valle RF, Sciarra JJ. Intrauterine adhesions: hysteroscopic diagnosis, classification, treatment, and reproductive outcome. Am J Obstet Gynecol. 1988;158:1459–70.
7. Donnez J, Nisolle M. Hysteroscopic lysis of intrauterine adhesions (Asherman syndrome). In: Donnez J, editor. Atlas of laser operative laparoscopy and hysteroscopy. New York, NY: Press-Parthenon; 1994. p. 305–22.
8. The American Fertility Society. Classifications of adnexal adhesions, distal tubal occlusion, tubal occlusion secondary to tubal ligation, tubal pregnancies, mullerian anomalies and intrauterine adhesions. Fertil Steril. 1988;49:944–55.
9. Wamsteker K, De Blok SJ. Diagnostic hysteroscopy: technique and documentation. In: Sutton C, Diamon M, editors. Endoscopic surgery for gynecologists. New York: Lippincott Williams & Wilkins Publishers; 1995. p. 263–76.
10. Nasr AL, Al-Inany H, Thabet S, Aboulghar M. A clinicohysteroscopic scoring system of intrauterine adhesions. Gynecol Obstet Investig. 2000;50:178–81.

11. Chithra S, Manchanda R, Jain N, Lekhi A. Role of hysteroscopy in diagnosis of Asherman's syndrome: a retrospective study. Int J Curr Res. 2016;8(5):31963–70.
12. Sharma R, Manchanda R, Chandil N. Revisiting diagnostic and therapeutic challenges in Asherman's syndrome: a retrospective analysis of 5 years. Int J Curr Res. 2018;10(8):72429–34.
13. AAGL Elevating Gynecologic Surgery. AAGL practice report: practice guidelines on intrauterine adhesions developed in collaboration with the European Society of Gynaecological Endoscopy (ESGE). J Minim Invasive Gynecol. 2017;24(5):695–705. https://doi.org/10.1016/j.jmig.2016.11.008.

Diagnosis: Patient Evaluation (Flowchart)

5

Antonio Simone Laganà, Simone Garzon, Gaetano Riemma, and Salvatore Giovanni Vitale

5.1 Introduction

The diagnosis of intrauterine adhesions (IUAs) and Asherman's syndrome has always been challenging [1, 2]. To date, the development of diagnostic techniques and the raised awareness of the condition have led to a more reliable diagnosis and management of this intrauterine pathology [3].

Hysteroscopy has been recognized as the gold standard for both the diagnosis and treatment of intrauterine adhesions, allowing clear visualization of the uterine cavity [4–8]. Nevertheless, the correct diagnostic flowchart (Fig. 5.1) for both IUAs and Asherman's syndrome should start from clinical suspicion and ultrasonography and, therefore, confirmation by hysteroscopy or, when hysteroscopy is not available, by other diagnostic techniques such as hysterosalpingography (HSG), sonohysterography (SHG), or magnetic resonance imaging (MRI) [1].

5.1.1 Clinical Suspicion

IUAs can be asymptomatic or symptomatic [3]. Usually, women can refer no symptoms as well as menstrual disorders, including infrequent, mild, or no

A. S. Laganà (✉) · S. Garzon
Department of Obstetrics and Gynecology, "Filippo Del Ponte" Hospital, University of Insubria, Varese, Italy
e-mail: antoniosimone.lagana@uninsubria.it

G. Riemma
Department of Women, Child, and General and Specialized Surgery, University of Campania "Luigi Vanvitelli", Naples, Italy

S. G. Vitale
Unit of Gynecology and Obstetrics, Department of General Surgery and Medical Surgical Specialties, University of Catania, Catania, Italy

R. Manchanda (ed.), *Intra Uterine Adhesions*,
https://doi.org/10.1007/978-981-33-4145-6_5

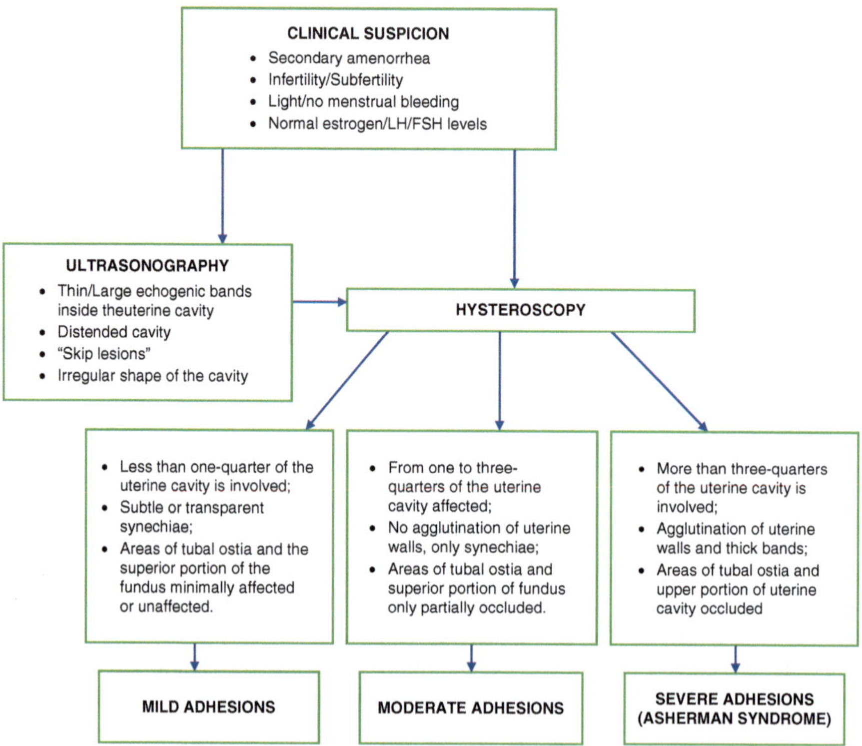

Fig. 5.1 Flowchart for the diagnosis of intrauterine adhesions and Asherman's syndrome

bleeding, reduced days of menstruation, dysmenorrhea, and, very rarely, heavy menstrual bleeding [9, 10]. In particular, menstrual bleeding is not strictly linked to the severity and location of adhesions [11]. Patients could complain of secondary infertility as the initial symptom, which is associated with Asherman's syndrome in approximately 40% of women [12]. In this regard, it has been hypothesized that disturbed endometrial vascularization, due to adhesions, could lead to implantation failure; in addition, embryo implantation could be impaired due to mechanical impediments (partially or totally obliterated uterine cavity) [13].

The vaginal examination does not provide reliable information regarding the potential presence of IUAs, so the diagnosis should rely first of all on an accurate and detailed clinical history collection to rule out other possible causes of secondary amenorrhea/hypomenorrhea/menstrual irregularities and/or infertility, as well as identify risk factors for IUAs such as intrauterine curettage, uterine embolization, B-lynch sutures, abdominal/hysteroscopic myomectomy, genital tuberculosis, or surgical treatment of Müllerian anomalies [14–21]. After clinical history collection, ultrasonography represents the first step to investigate IUAs.

5.1.2 Ultrasonography

Ultrasonography should be used routinely as the first diagnostic tool, although the skill of the operator affects the diagnostic accuracy of the technique [22]. Intrauterine adhesions can be focused as transversal bands of myometrial tissue that cross the uterine cavity and connect the opposing uterine walls. Usually, bands have the same or augmented echogenicity of the surrounding myometrium and vary in length and thickness [23].

In the case of mild adhesions, endometrium should be clearly visible, and thin echogenic bands should be visualized inside a distended uterine cavity. The more the syndrome is severe, the most the bands should be rigid and thick, with hypoechogenic material between them. In the case of severe adhesions, the uterine cavity could be found morphologically irregular with a loss of endometrial echo [24].

A typical endometrial pattern is represented by "skip lesions": interruptions of the endometrial layer by means of several hypoechoic areas, which are images of accumulated menstrual blood or detached endometrium [9].

The operator should be aware that if the internal cervical orifice is obliterated, the uterine cavity may be distended by menstrual blood and debris. Transversal bands are often not visible [22]. In case of significant IUAs, the endometrium could appear thin (atrophic) because of low estrogenic responsiveness that usually is restored after IUA divisions [22].

Nevertheless, data published so far are not robust enough to lead to an agreement about the sensitivity of ultrasonography for the diagnosis of IUAs and Asherman's syndrome [25, 26]. To date, although the evolution of 3D and 4D ultrasonography has somehow improved the diagnostic accuracy with respect to the "classic" 2D scan [27, 28], further trials are needed to assess their efficacy in terms of sensitivity, specificity, and positive and negative predictive values.

5.1.3 Hysteroscopy

Hysteroscopy is a feasible, safe, and cost-effective diagnostic and therapeutic option for IUAs and Asherman's syndrome [29–32]. During hysteroscopy, adhesions can be generally described in several ways: thin or subtle bands or stripes without vascularization that connect two opposite walls, or agglutinations of the walls that are able to completely or partially obliterate the uterine cavity [22]. It is essential for the operator to carefully define the number, location, extension, and structure of adhesions, as follows:

A. **Number**: the number of synechiae inside the cavity
B. **Location of adhesions**: central or marginal
    B1. Central: columnar shaped bands attached to two opposite walls of the uterine cavity with blazed ends
    B2. Marginal: sickle-shaped bands able to obliterate the uterine wall partially; the uterine cavity appears asymmetrical in shape

C. **Extension:** mild, moderate, or severe

If the synechiae completely obliterate the cavity, this appears narrow and assumes a tubular-shaped conformation. In the case of Asherman's syndrome (severe synechiae in association with dysmenorrhea and changes in menstrual patterns), only fibrous tissue could be seen, with just poor irregular endometrial bridges linked in between.

D. **Structure and consistency:** identify which tissue is predominant (mucosal, muscular, or fibrous)

D1. Mucosal: similar to the healthy physiological endometrium, easy to resect, delicate, laminar, without vascularization or specific structure.

D2. Muscular: structured with an axis of muscular tissue covered by a thin line of endometrium surrounded by glandular outlets.

D3. Fibrous: those synechiae are composed primarily of connective tissue, which can be easily differentiated from normal endometrium; they appear white and translucent, with no vascularization and mainly surrounded by atrophic endometrium.

It is important for the operator to schematically categorize adhesions using a specific classification system. To date, several classification systems are being routinely used by gynecologists [29–31, 33, 34]; however, there is no evidence supporting the superiority of one over the others [1]. The first classification was developed by March et al. in 1978 [29]. This classification divides IUAs into three groups according to extension in mild, moderate, and severe (Table 5.1). Among the other classification systems, there are those developed by Valle and Sciarra in 1988 [31], by Donnez and Nisolle in 1994 [35], and by the American Fertility Society in 1998 [34], which is to date the most used worldwide.

5.1.4 Other Diagnostic Techniques

HSG using contrast dye has a sensitivity of 75–81%, a specificity of 80%, and a positive predictive value of 50% compared to hysteroscopy for diagnosis of IUAs [22, 26, 36]. Using HSG, synechiae were indirectly referred to as filling defects and

Table 5.1 Classification of intrauterine adhesions developed by March et al. (1978)

Classes	Hysteroscopic appearance
Mild	• Less than one-quarter of the uterine cavity is involved; subtle or transparent synechiae; areas of tubal ostia and the superior portion of the fundus minimally affected or unaffected
Moderate	• From one- to three-quarters of the uterine cavity affected • No agglutination of uterine walls, only synechiae • Areas of tubal ostia and superior portion of fundus only partially occluded
Severe	• More than three-quarters of the uterine cavity is involved (Asherman's syndrome) • Agglutination of uterine walls and thick bands • Areas of tubal ostia and upper portion of uterine cavity occluded

irregularly in-between-shaped spaces in images, with clear margins and homogeneous opacity. When severe IUAs are suspected, the uterine cavity would appear reduced in volume and distorted in shape with occluded tubes in the majority of cases [37]. Compared to hysteroscopy, HSG has been reported to have a similar sensitivity, although a large number of false-positive findings are considered a limitation to its use [26, 36].

SHG, also called saline infusion sonography (SIS) or gel infusion sonography (GIS), was found to be as effective as HSG, with both reported to have a sensitivity of 75% and a positive predictive value of 43% for SHG or SIS/GIS and 50% for HSG, compared to hysteroscopy [26, 38].

MRI has also been evaluated for the diagnosis of IUAs; nevertheless, the high cost of the procedure does not justify its routine use for diagnosis of IUAs and Asherman's syndrome [39, 40].

Key Points

1. Secondary infertility as an initial symptom is associated with Asherman's syndrome in approximately 40% of women.
2. Menstrual disorders, such as mild or no bleeding, reduced days of menstruations, and dysmenorrhea, could also be associated.
3. The most common risk factors for Asherman's syndrome are previous intrauterine curettage, uterine embolization, B-lynch sutures, abdominal/hysteroscopic myomectomy, genital tuberculosis, or surgical treatment of Müllerian anomalies.
4. The vaginal examination does not provide reliable diagnostic information for Asherman's syndrome.
5. After an initial assessment by medical history, an ultrasound scan should be considered the first diagnostic step.
6. At the ultrasound scan, intrauterine adhesions can be focused as transversal bands of myometrial tissue that cross the uterine cavity and connect the opposing uterine walls. Usually, bands have the same or increased echogenicity of the surrounding myometrium and can vary in length and thickness.
7. The more the syndrome is severe, the most the bands should be rigid and thick, with hypoechogenic material between them. In the case of severe adhesions, the uterine cavity could be found morphologically irregular with a loss of endometrial echoes.
8. After an ultrasound scan, the confirmation of Asherman's syndrome is recommended by hysteroscopy, describing the following elements: number, location, extension, structure, and consistency of adhesions.
9. To date, there is no evidence supporting the use of one classification system of intrauterine adhesions over the others, although the most used worldwide was developed by the American Fertility Society.
10. Magnetic resonance imaging is not cost-effective for the diagnosis of intrauterine adhesions.

References

1. Dreisler E, Kjer JJ. Asherman's syndrome: current perspectives on diagnosis and management. Int J Women's Health. 2019;20:191–9.
2. Zupi E, Centini G, Lazzeri L. Asherman syndrome: an unsolved clinical definition and management. Fertil Steril. 2015;104:1380–1.
3. Hanstede MMF, Van Der Meij E, Goedemans L, Emanuel MH. Results of centralized Asherman surgery, 2003–2013. Fertil Steril. 2015;104:1561.e1–8.e1.
4. Khan Z, Goldberg JM. Hysteroscopic management of Asherman's syndrome. J Minim Invasive Gynecol. 2018;25:218–28.
5. Bougie O, Lortie K, Shenassa H, Chen I, Singh SS. Treatment of Asherman's syndrome in an outpatient hysteroscopy setting. J Minim Invasive Gynecol. 2015;22:446–50.
6. Amer-Cuenca JJ, Marín-Buck A, Vitale SG, La Rosa VL, Caruso S, Cianci A, Lisón JF. Nonpharmacological pain control in outpatient hysteroscopies. Minim Invasive Ther Allied Technol. 2020;29(1):10–9. https://doi.org/10.1080/13645706.2019.1576054.
7. Kriseman M, Schutt A, Appleton J, Pillai A, George V, Zarutskie PW. A novel ultrasound-guided technique for hysteroscopic adhesiolysis in high-risk patients. J Ultrasound Med. 2019;38:1383–7.
8. Laganà AS, Vitale SG, Muscia V, et al. Endometrial preparation with dienogest before hysteroscopic surgery: a systematic review. Arch Gynecol Obstet. 2017;295:661–7.
9. Yu D, Wong YM, Cheong Y, Xia E, Li TC. Asherman syndrome - one century later. Fertil Steril. 2008;89:759–79.
10. Salazar CA, Isaacson K, Morris S. A comprehensive review of Asherman's syndrome: causes, symptoms and treatment options. Curr Opin Obstet Gynecol. 2017;29:249–56.
11. March CM. Management of Asherman's syndrome. Reprod BioMed Online. 2011;23:63–76.
12. Tsui KH, Te Lin L, Cheng JT, Teng SW, Wang PH. Comprehensive treatment for infertile women with severe Asherman syndrome. Taiwan J Obstet Gynecol. 2014;53:372–5.
13. Azizi R, Aghebati-Maleki L, Nouri M, Marofi F, Negargar S, Yousefi M. Stem cell therapy in Asherman syndrome and thin endometrium: stem cell-based therapy. Biomed Pharmacother. 2018;102:333–43.
14. Song D, Liu Y, Xiao Y, Li TC, Zhou F, Xia E. A matched cohort study comparing the outcome of intrauterine adhesiolysis for Asherman's syndrome after uterine artery embolization or surgical trauma. J Minim Invasive Gynecol. 2014;21(6):1022–8. https://doi.org/10.1016/j.jmig.2014.04.015.
15. Vitale SG, Sapia F, Rapisarda AMC, et al. Hysteroscopic morcellation of submucous myomas: a systematic review. Biomed Res Int. 2017;2017:6848250.
16. Zhu R, Gan L, Wang S, Duan H. A cohort study comparing the severity and outcome of intrauterine adhesiolysis for Asherman syndrome after first- or second-trimester termination of pregnancy. Eur J Obstet Gynecol Reprod Biol. 2019;238:49–53.
17. Gilman Barber AR, Rhone SA, Fluker MR. Curettage and Asherman's syndrome-lessons to (re-) learn? J Obstet Gynaecol Can. 2014;36:997–1001.
18. Di Spiezio SA, Gencarelli A, Vieira MDC, Riemma G, De Simone T, Carugno J. Differentiating a rare uterine lipoleiomyoma from uterine perforation at hysteroscopy: a scary story. J Minim Invasive Gynecol. 2019;27(1):9–10. https://doi.org/10.1016/j.jmig.2019.04.020.
19. Laganà AS, Alonso Pacheco L, Tinelli A, Haimovich S, Carugno J, Ghezzi F, Mazzon I, Bettocchi S. Management of asymptomatic submucous myomas in women of reproductive age: a consensus statement from the global congress on hysteroscopy scientific committee. J Minim Invasive Gynecol. 2019;26:381–3.
20. Alonso Pacheco L, Laganà AS, Ghezzi F, Haimovich S, Azumendi Gómez P, Carugno J. Subtypes of T-shaped uterus. Fertil Steril. 2019;112:399–400.
21. Alonso Pacheco L, Laganà AS, Garzon S, Perez Garrido A, Flores Gornes A, Ghezzi F. Hysteroscopic outpatient metroplasty for T-shaped uterus in women with reproductive

failure: results from a large prospective cohort study. Eur J Obstet Gynecol Reprod Biol. 2019;243:173–8. https://doi.org/10.1016/j.ejogrb.2019.09.023.

22. Amin TN, Saridogan E, Jurkovic D. Ultrasound and intrauterine adhesions: a novel structured approach to diagnosis and management. Ultrasound Obstet Gynecol. 2015;46:131–9.
23. Leone FPG, Timmerman D, Bourne T, et al. Terms, definitions and measurements to describe the sonographic features of the endometrium and intrauterine lesions: a consensus opinion from the International Endometrial Tumor Analysis (IETA) group. Ultrasound Obstet Gynecol. 2010;35:103–12.
24. Naftalin J, Jurkovic D. The endometrial-myometrial junction: a fresh look at a busy crossing. Ultrasound Obstet Gynecol. 2009;34:1–11.
25. Fedele L, Bianchi S, Dorta M, Vignali M. Intrauterine adhesions: detection with transvaginal US. Radiology. 1996;199:757–9.
26. Soares SR, Dos Reis MMBB, Camargos AF. Diagnostic accuracy of sonohysterography, transvaginal sonography, and hysterosalpingography in patients with uterine cavity diseases. Fertil Steril. 2000;73:406–11.
27. Knopman J, Copperman AB. Value of 3D ultrasound in the management of suspected Asherman's syndrome. J Reprod Med Obstet Gynecol. 2007;52:1016–22.
28. Laganà AS, Ciancimino L, Mancuso A, Chiofalo B, Rizzo P, Triolo O. 3D sonohysterography vs. hysteroscopy: a cross-sectional study for the evaluation of endouterine diseases. Arch Gynecol Obstet. 2014;290:1173–8.
29. March CM, Israel R, March AD. Hysteroscopic management of intrauterine adhesions. Am J Obstet Gynecol. 1978;130:653–7.
30. Hamou J, Cittadini E, Perino A. Diagnosis and management of intrauterine adhesions by microhysteroscopy. Acta Eur Fertil. 1983;14:117–23.
31. Valle RF, Sciarra JJ. Intrauterine adhesions: hysteroscopic diagnosis, classification, treatment, and reproductive outcome. Am J Obstet Gynecol. 1988;158:1459–70.
32. Pabuçcu R, Urman B, Atay V, Ergün A, Orhon E. Hysteroscopic treatment of intrauterine adhesions is safe and effective in the restoration of normal menstruation and fertility. Fertil Steril. 1997;68:1141–3.
33. Aboul Nasr AL, Al-Inany HG, Thabet SM, Aboulghar M. A clinicohysteroscopic scoring system of intrauterine adhesions. Gynecol Obstet Investig. 2000;50:178–81.
34. Buttram VC, Gomel V, Siegler A, DeCherney A, Gibbons W, March C. The American Fertility Society classifications of adnexal adhesions, distal tubal occlusion, tubal occlusion secondary to tubal ligation, tubal pregnancies, Mullerian anomalies and intrauterine adhesions. Fertil Steril. 1988;49:944–55.
35. Donnez J, Nisolle M. Hysteroscopic adhesiolysis of intrauterine adhesions (Asherman syndrome). Hysteroscopy: An Atlas Laser Oper. Laparosc; 1994.
36. Dalfó AR, Úbeda B, Úbeda A, Monzón M, Rotger R, Ramos R, Palacio A. Diagnostic value of hysterosalpingography in the detection of intrauterine abnormalities: a comparison with hysteroscopy. Am J Roentgenol. 2004;183:1405–9.
37. Ahmadi F, Siahbazi S, Akhbari F, Eslami B, Vosough A. Hysterosalpingography finding in intrauterine adhesion (Asherman's syndrome): a pictorial essay. Int J Fertil Steril. 2013;7:155–60.
38. Salle B, Gaucherand P, De Saint Hilaire P, Rudigoz RC. Transvaginal sonohysterographic evaluation of intrauterine adhesions. J Clin Ultrasound. 1999;27:131–4.
39. Letterie GS, Haggerty MF. Magnetic resonance imaging of intrauterine synechiae. Gynecol Obstet Investig. 1994;37:66–8.
40. Bacelar AC, Wilcock D, Powell M, Worthington BS. The value of MRI in the assessment of traumatic intra-uterine adhesions (Asherman's syndrome). Clin Radiol. 1995;50:80–3.

Ultrasound Diagnosis and Management 6

Ashok Khurana

Since the pioneering publications of Fritsch [1] and Asherman [2, 3] the understanding and management of intrauterine adhesions (IUAs) have come a long way [4–11].

The criteria for the "syndrome" have been expanded beyond the original "secondary amenorrhea." The term "Asherman syndrome" is currently loosely used. The original term referred to obliterative or obstructive IUAs with pain, menstrual disturbances, and subfertility in any combination. It now includes all conditions of partial or complete obliteration or obstruction of the uterine cavity where a patient may present with a spectrum of clinical manifestations including no symptoms, amenorrhea, oligomenorrhea, hypomenorrhea, cyclical pain, infertility, recurrent pregnancy loss, fetal malpresentations in pregnancy, low-lying placenta, or invasive placenta [5, 6, 12].

6.1 Synonyms for IUAs

The term "intrauterine adhesions" is interchangeably used with "intrauterine synechiae." Older nomenclature included "uterine atresia" and "endometrial sclerosis."

6.2 Etiology of IUAs

The etiology of synechiae in the cavity has some bearing on the morphology of the cavity on ultrasound and some specific pointers including those seen in tubercular disease [13, 14]. These are described later in this chapter.

A. Khurana (✉)
The Ultrasound Lab, New Delhi, India
e-mail: ashokkhurana@ashokkhurana.com

R. Manchanda (ed.), *Intra Uterine Adhesions*,
https://doi.org/10.1007/978-981-33-4145-6_6

6.3 Classification of IUAs

Several major classifications [12, 15–17] are widely used for describing lesions and have no consensus [18, 19]. These are based on hysteroscopic and hysterosalpingographic findings and do not incorporate ultrasound findings. The European Society of Hysteroscopy (ESH) system distinguishes stages based on adhesion band thickness, tubal ostia patency, and degree of uterine cavity obliteration on direct visualization. The American Society for Reproductive Medicine (ASRM) includes menstrual pattern, potentially offering some prognostic information. Unfortunately, the categories do not coincide with the wide variety of morphology evident on ultrasound images today. Surgical experts and imaging experts are on different pages and this is of no benefit to the patient. This treatise attempts to bridge that gap.

6.4 Pathologic Basis of Symptoms and Imaging

Stromal loss consequent to endometrial injury is the essential event leading to the formation of IUAs. Fibrous tissue replaces areas of lost stroma and this causes apposing endometrial surfaces to stick together, resulting in the formation of IUAs. Delineation between the functional and basal layers of the endometrium is obliterated [11]. Both these layers are replaced by an atrophic epithelial monolayer that is avascular and does not respond to cyclical or therapeutic hormonal influences [4].

A knowledge of the possible cause for IUAs in a given patient serves as a guide for good imaging. For example, a previous cesarean section can induce adhesions superior to the cervix (Fig. 6.1a, b) and this region should be specifically observed. The 2D image fails to show most of the features.

In the background of a previous ectopic pregnancy or tuberculosis, distortion of the normal configuration of the ostial aspects of the cavity needs to be specifically

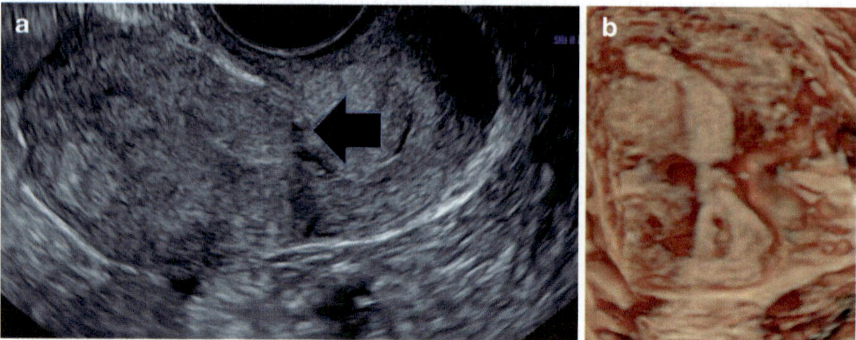

Fig. 6.1 (**a**) Note the cesarean scar (arrow) and the interruption of the endometrium at this level and in the entire corpus, except the fundal region in the routine 2D image. (**b**) Shows interruption of the endometrium at the level of the scar, the hemi-uterus (unicornuate) configuration, synechiae in the endocervix, and a diffuse irregularity and narrowing of the uterine cavity in the 3D image

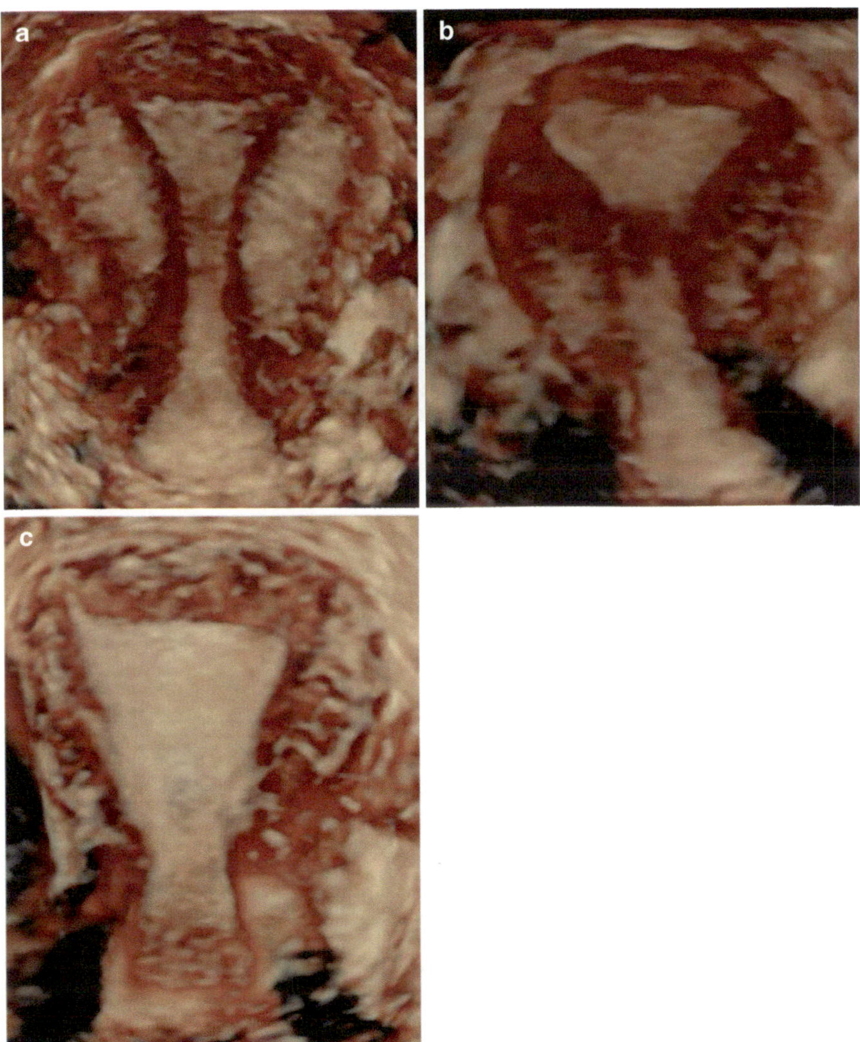

Fig. 6.2 (**a**) A normal 3D cavity. (**b**) Shows amputation of the ostial ends of the cavity on both sides. Note also synechiae causing absence of echoes superior to the cervix. (**c**) Shows a vertical course of the interstitial course of the right tube, a reliable indicator of tuberculosis

delineated. This is best done with 3D technology, and therefore this should be available on the equipment used for ultrasound (Fig. 6.2a–c).

IUAs can be focal, partial, complete, obstructive, or obliterative [11] and this should guide the protocol to be followed for an exhaustive evaluation by ultrasound or hysterosalpingograms. Obstructive symptoms need delineation of fluid in the cavity and this will be best seen during the menstrual phase of the cycle (Fig. 6.3).

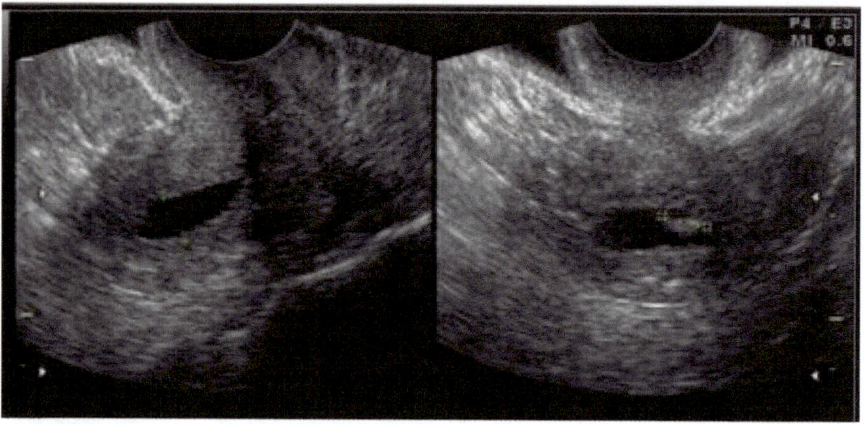

Fig. 6.3 Menstrual fluid in the cavity outlining a synechiae

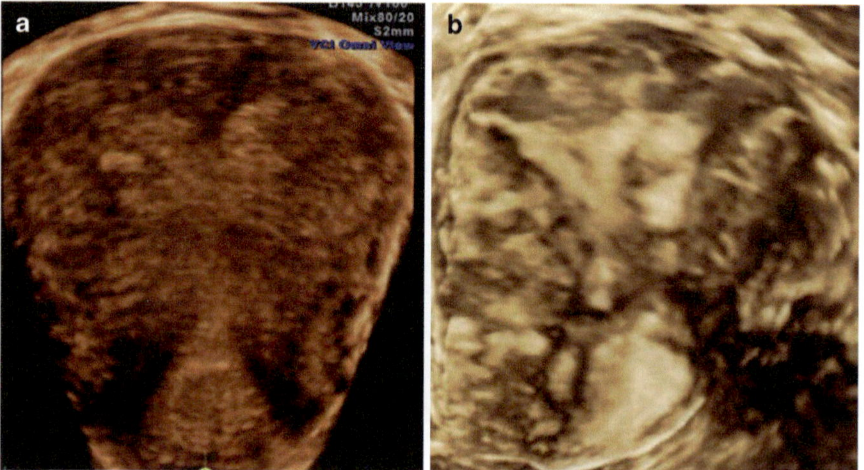

Fig. 6.4 (**a**) Shows scanty interrupted endometrium, assessed on cycle day 6. (**b**) Secretory-phase study shows a far greater extent of residual endometrium

The extent of adhesions and the presence of residual functioning endometrium have major implications on treatment options, surgical goals, and patient outcomes. This can be assessed and quantified on 3D ultrasound. The extent of residual endometrium will be better assessed in the mid-cycle or secretory phase of the cycle (Fig. 6.4a, b).

Extensive obliteration of the cavity is best studied by 3D reconstruction, 3D rotation, and 3D multislice imaging [11] (Fig. 6.5a–c).

If obstructive symptoms are prominent and 2D and 3D ultrasounds do not reveal adhesions, the examination should be extended to include a fluid/gel infusion sonohysterography (Fig. 6.6).

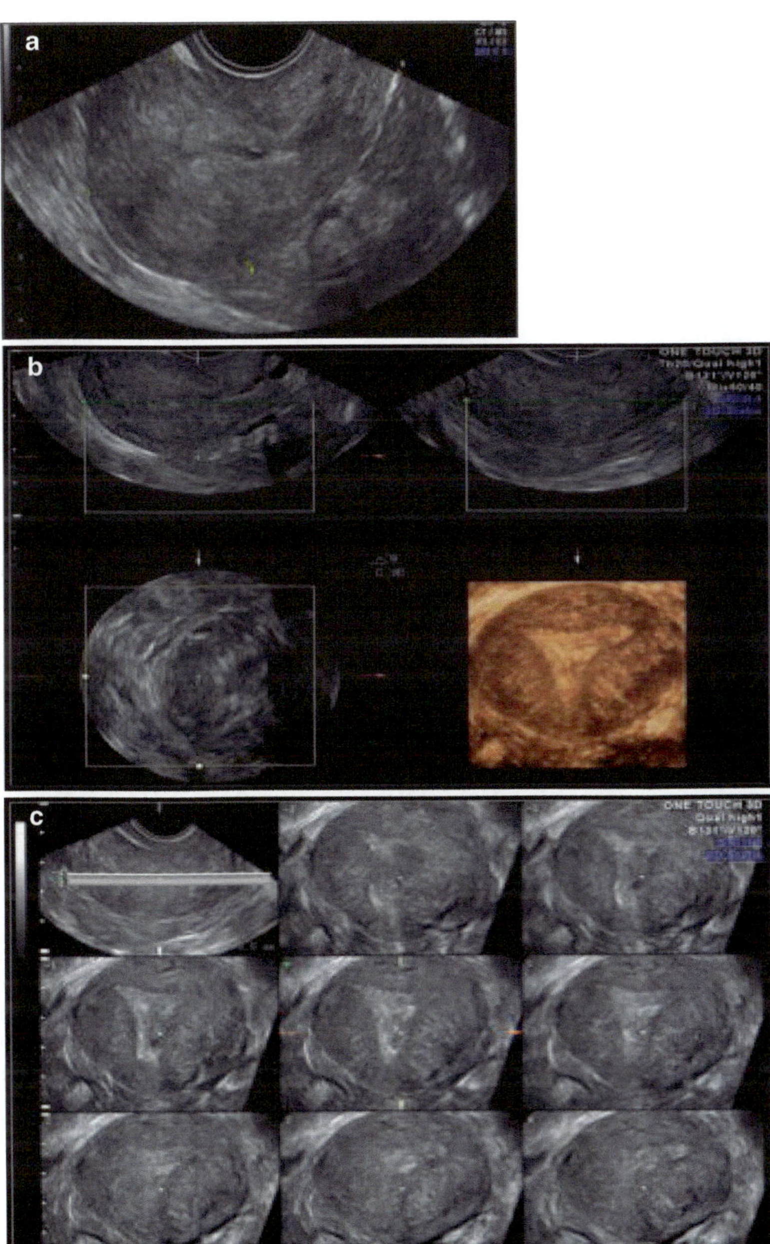

Fig. 6.5 (**a**) Shows a 2D image of a thin endometrium. (**b**) Shows a 3D multiplanar display of the same patient with a coronal rendering of the cavity. Note the poorly defined interrupted endometrium. (**c**) The 3D reconstruction is displayed in a multislice format as in CT and MRI scans. The slices are in the coronal plane and are parallel. They are closely placed over the entire extent of the endometrium. Note the multiple interruptions of the cavity almost obliterating it. The extent of obliteration is best understood by studying the entire extent of the endometrium in the multislice format

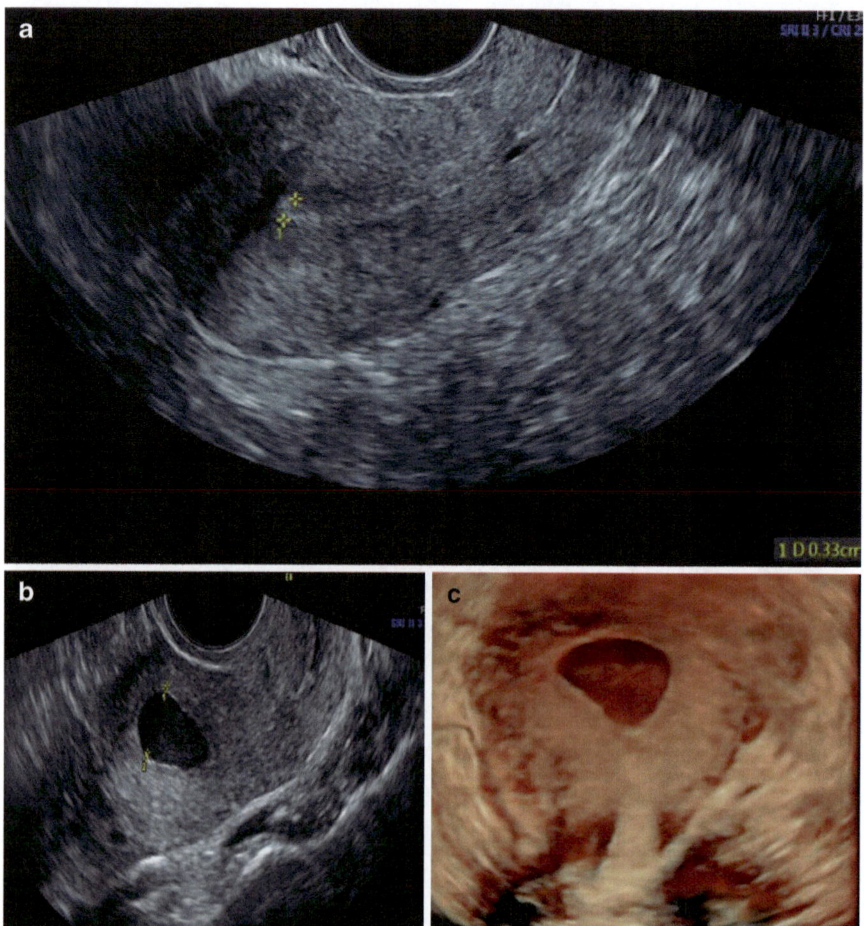

Fig. 6.6 (**a**) Evaluation of a patient with secondary amenorrhea and cyclical pain. A 2D evaluation reveals a thin endometrium. (**b**) Saline infusion sonography shows accumulation of fluid in the uterine cavity. Careful inspection reveals the collection stopping short in the midcorpus. The cavity in the lower part of the cavity is completely obliterated by scarring. (**c**) Note how it is easier to appreciate this in the 3D coronal format (**c**) compared to the 2D sagittal format

6.5 Diagnostic Options in Perspective

Asherman syndrome cannot be diagnosed by a routine gynecological physical examination [20, 21]. Introducing a uterine sound may reveal obstruction at or near the internal os [21]. Sounding of the uterus cannot assess adhesions in the mid and upper parts of the corpus and those that are located on the lateral aspect of the cavity. Hysteroscopy has been established as the gold standard for diagnosis of IUAs [11, 12, 15, 16]. Provided that the uterine cavity is accessible, hysteroscopy is more accurate than radiological imaging techniques [8, 11, 12].

Hysteroscopy is superior in assessing the presence or absence of adhesions, morphological features of adhesions, and quality of residual endometrium. It enables classification of IUAs [22] and concurrent treatment. It must be noted, however, that the reproducibility of hysteroscopy is questionable because it relies completely on the subjective impression of the performing operator [23].

Several considerations necessitate the need for pre-hysteroscopic imaging. The first consideration is the rare but known risk of an invasive procedure under general anesthesia in any patient. The second risk to be kept in perspective is perforation of the uterus. Additionally, the success of hysteroscopy depends entirely upon the accessibility of the uterine cavity.

Imaging can warn of possible obstruction just beyond the internal os and to a large extent the rest of the cavity, and this can greatly contribute to diagnostic and operative success [24]. In patients with very extensive IUAs obliterating the lower part of the uterine cavity, hysteroscopy may fail because of inability to negotiate the lower part of the corpus and identify surgical planes. Ultrasound, in fact, is being increasingly used to access the cavity during anticipated difficult access [24].

The past decade has witnessed rapid changes in surgical instrumentation and operative technique and this demands as much of a presurgical morphological delineation in order to ensure availability of various instruments. Imaging greatly fulfills this need. Most patients expect to be given treatment options such as expectant management, trial of nonsurgical treatment, and fast-tracking to surgical options. Good imaging prior to hysteroscopy serves as a road map not only for access, type of procedure, instruments, and patient counseling but also for scheduling of surgeries and assessment of costs. Presurgical mapping of the uterine cavity can facilitate this. Infertile couples, too, expect a similar cafeteria approach including fast-tracking to fertility-enhancing surgery and surrogacy (Fig. 6.7a–f).

Imaging may also contribute to offering more appropriate cost estimations and efficient operating room scheduling.

Hysterosalpingography (HSG) has a 75–80% sensitivity and specificity for diagnosis of IUAs compared to hysteroscopy [25–28]. The positive predictive value, however, is 50% and the false-positive rate is 39% [25]. As in hysteroscopy, HSG frequently fails in patients with complete obstruction in or just above the cervix or when the cavity is extensively obliterated [4, 12]. These factors along with radiation exposure and invasiveness make the role of HSG questionable for the detection of IUAs, although it retains its place as a screening test in the infertile patient. Filling defects and an irregular cavity outline are the findings of IUAs on an HSG.

Sonohysterography (SHG) is an ultrasound procedure where saline, gel, or foam is instilled into the uterine cavity via the cervix. This is then also referred to as saline infusion sonography (SIS), saline infusion sonohysterography (SISH), gel infusion sonography (GIS), and foam infusion sonography. SHG has a sensitivity of about 75% and a positive predictive value of 43% for the detection of IUAs, compared to hysteroscopy. Because SHG is radiation free, does not require a radiology suite, and has similar sensitivity and positive predictive value as HSG, it has emerged as a convenient screening test for IUAs [29–36].

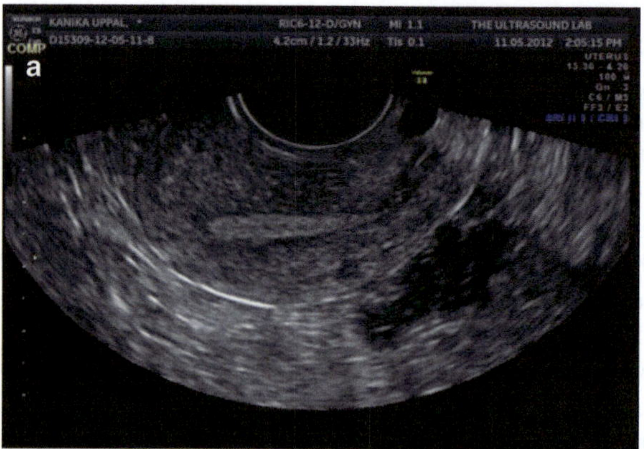

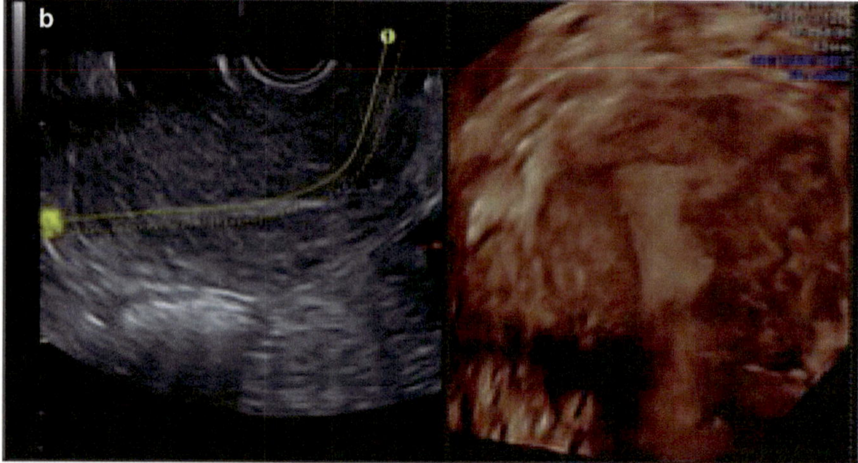

Fig. 6.7 (**a**) 2D image of a nonresponsive endometrium in an IVF case. Figure (**b**) shows 3D images of a nonresponsive endometrium in an IVF case. Note the lack of detail in the 2D image compared to the 3D reconstruction. The 3D image shows a potential block of hysteroscopic access superior to the cervix and the possible need for ultrasound guidance for negotiating this area to be able to access the cavity for a potential lateral metroplasty followed by an extra effort to prevent recurrence. Figure (**c**) is a similar case where the obliteration is more extensive and, because of the extensive obliteration along the right wall in the mid and upper parts of the corpus, the possibility of a failed metroplasty must be included in counseling. Figure (**d**) shows a patient with a completely obliterated cavity and no recognizable cavity contour. Counseling needs to include the option of fast-tracking to surrogacy or adoption. (**e**) Shows an unremarkable secretory endometrium in the secretory phase of the cycle on 2D assessment. (**f**) 3D coronal reconstruction of the same patient showing synechiae in the midcorpus and a T-shaped cavity. This is well known to be consequent to a myometrial and endometrial endarteritis of tuberculosis. Surgery would include not only synechiectomy but the option of a lateral metroplasty as well

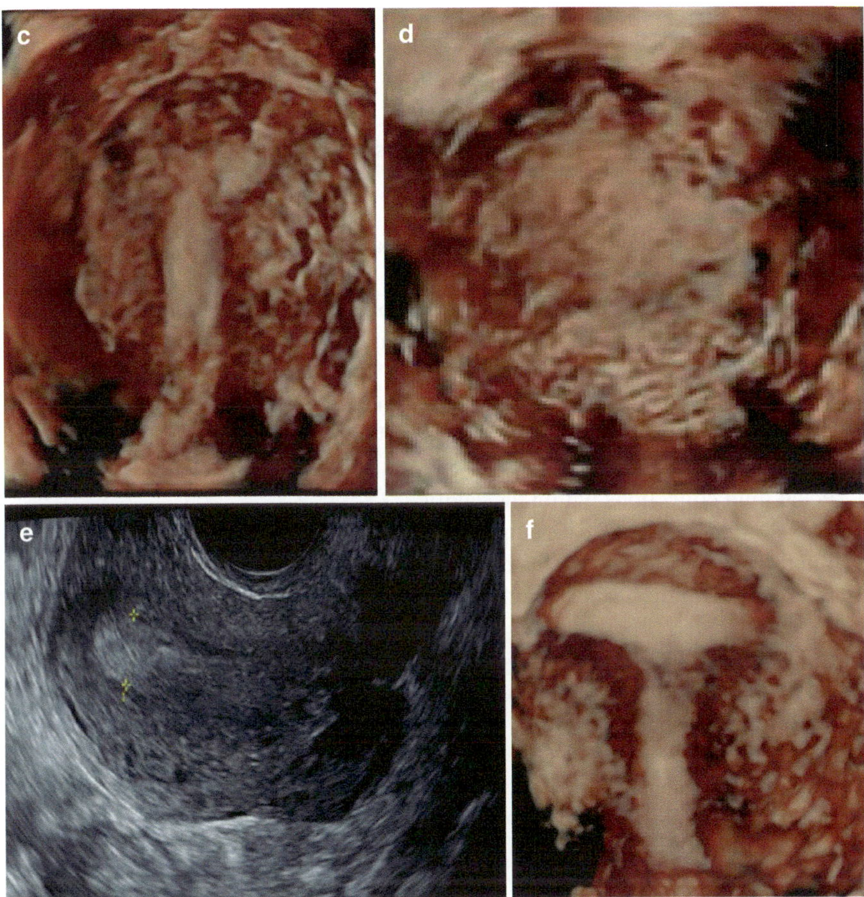

Fig. 6.7 (continued)

Routine 2D transvaginal ultrasound remains the mainstay for the preliminary search for IUAs not because of its statistical performance but because ultrasound is the first imaging technique to be performed on the patient after a routine physical examination. It has a reasonable sensitivity [29, 37], although an early study reported 0%. This study included only four patients. The evolution of technology and operator skill are known to remarkably affect accuracy [11, 38].

Three-dimensional (3D) ultrasound and 3D SHG have emerged as highly accurate techniques [11, 33, 38–41] for the evaluation of IUAs and are being increasingly regarded as "routine" in the management of IUAs.

Current assessments of magnetic resonance imaging (MRI) for the diagnosis of IUAs show no advantages over less expensive alternatives [42–45].

6.6 An Illustrated Guide to Imaging of IUAs

Ultrasound findings in IUAs include the following observations, singly or in combination. Figures 6.8, 6.9, 6.10, 6.11, 6.12, 6.13, 6.14, 6.15, and 6.16 illustrate these findings with extensive descriptions of findings and techniques:

- Thin, interrupted endometrium.
- Thin endometrium, nonresponsive to cyclical variation.
- Variably thinned endometrium.
- Interruptions in the continuity of the endometrium: These may be solitary or multiple, thick or thin, focal or extensive, and vascular or avascular.
- Cornual amputation of the cavity.
- Vertical course of the interstitial extent of the Fallopian tube.
- Irregular contour of the uterine cavity: focal, multiple, or extensive.
- Tubular configuration of the cavity.
- Focal fluid collections within the cavity.
- Free fluid in the cavity with a thin endometrium.
- Bands across the cavity outlined by instilled fluid/gel.
- Indirect indicators such as endometrial or subendometrial calcification, focal hyper-echogenicities without distal shadowing, and loss of endometrial/myometrial delineation.
- These findings may be evident on 2D, 3D, or fluid instillation studies.
- A normal ultrasound scan does not exclude intrauterine adhesions.

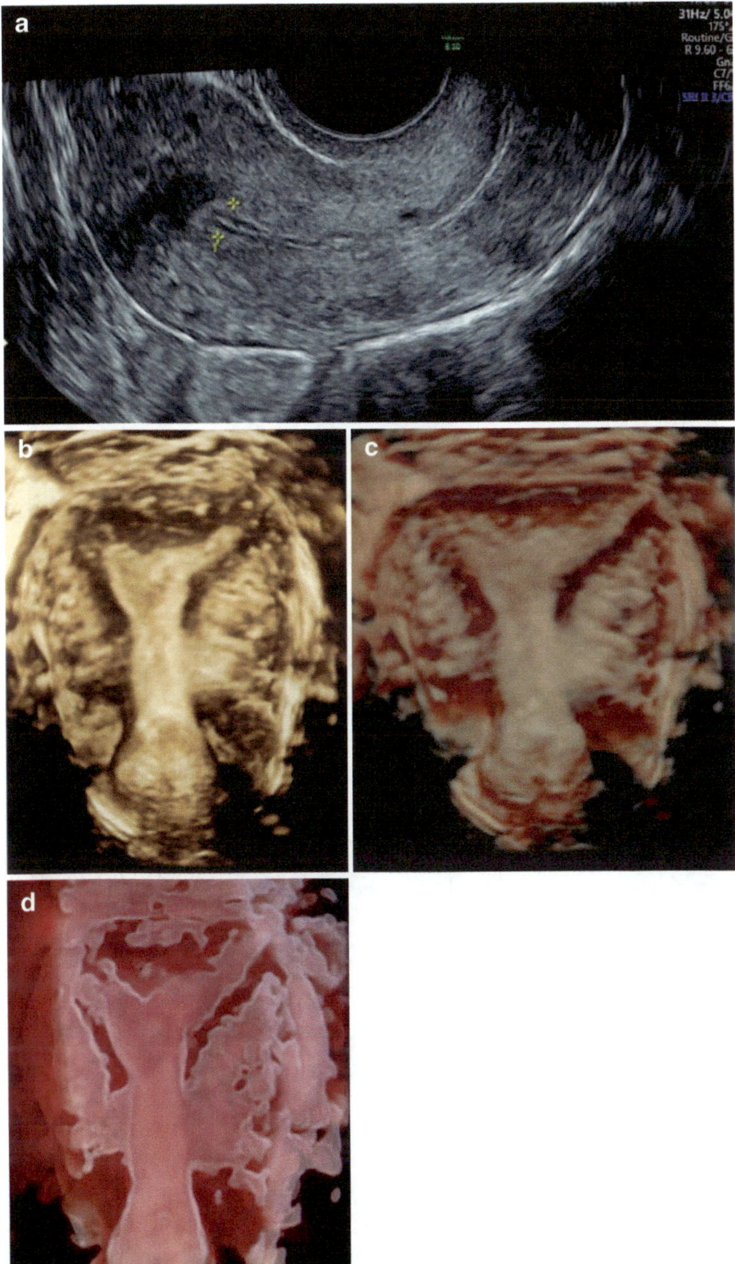

Fig. 6.8 (**a**) Shows an unremarkable early proliferative phase triple-layered endometrium. (**b**) 3D coronal reconstruction reveals additional information of a shallow fundal septum, a T-shaped cavity with a limited transverse extent, and obliteration of the right ostial extent of the cavity. (**c**) Using a newer 3D rendering engine and a software that enhances outlines (silhouette mode). (**d**) Delineates all aspects of the disease process with greater clarity and diagnostic confidence

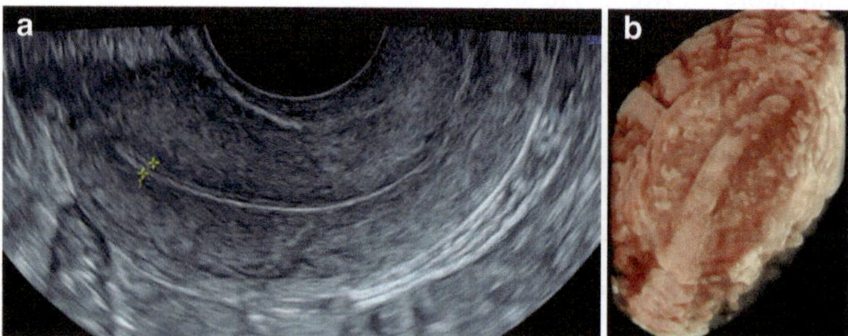

Fig. 6.9 (**a**) 2D evaluation largely fails to delineate Mullerian anomalies and IUAs. (**b**) Shows hemi-uterus (unicornuate of the older classifications) and extensive interruptions of the cavity representing IUAs. 3D is a rapid and efficient way to delineate both these conditions

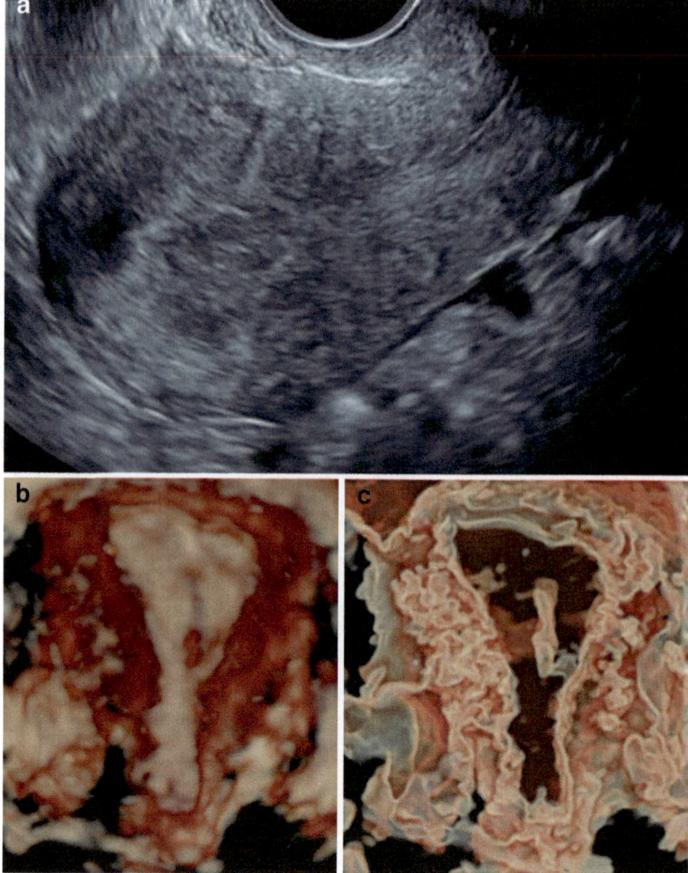

Fig. 6.10 (**a**) Shows 2D evaluation of irregularly marginated thick endometrium. (**b**) 3D USG. (**c**) Fluid infusion hysterography. (**b**, **c**) Because 3D does not carry the risk of reducing or disseminating infection, and is now widely available at a lesser cost, it becomes the appropriate choice. 3D evaluation in this case reveals thick IUAs and an irregular cavity contour. Both features were addressed during patient counseling, surgery, and postoperative protocols that may prevent a recurrence

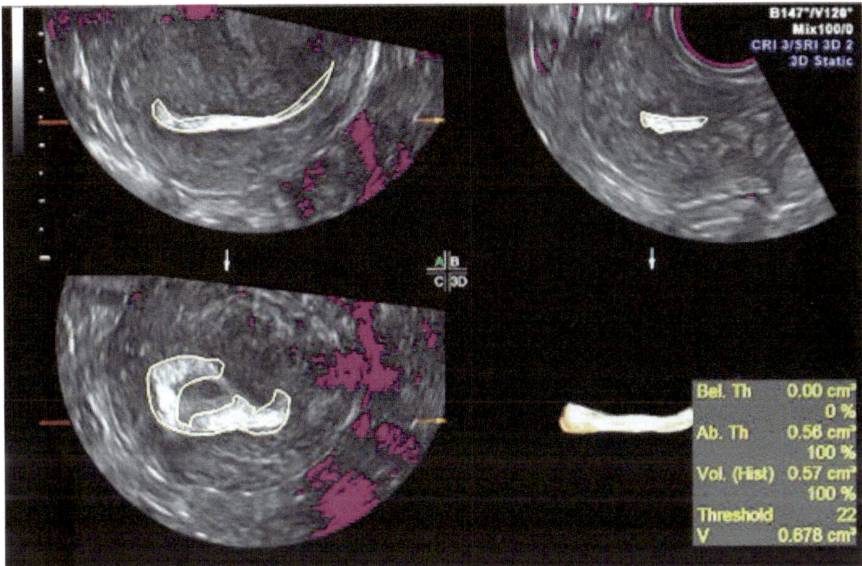

Fig. 6.11 As the endometrium thickens in response to medication or in a natural cycle, residual endometrium becomes more echogenic and IUAs remain hypoechoic. Volume calculation software permits measurement of functioning endometrium. Even with a poor and variable endometrial thickness, an adequate residual functional endometrial volume can support implantation

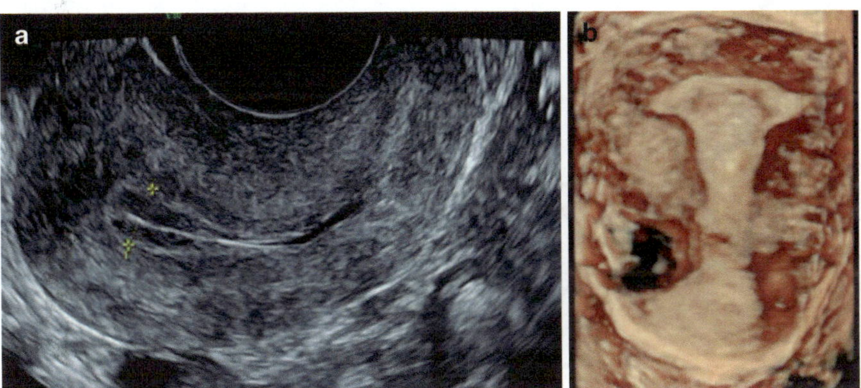

Fig. 6.12 (**a**) Shows fluid in the cavity on day 11 of a monitored ovulation cycle, prompting a search for IUAs. Irrespective of a normal proliferative morphology endometrium and an acceptable endometrial thickness, the presence of fluid in the uterine cavity must prompt a search for Asherman. (**b**) Shows 3D low-volume endometrium and multiple subtle interruptions of echo intensity in the cavity, confirming IUAs and a suboptimal endometrium. Volume casts and calculations have a steep learning curve and are easy to achieve after a minimum number of repetitions under supervision

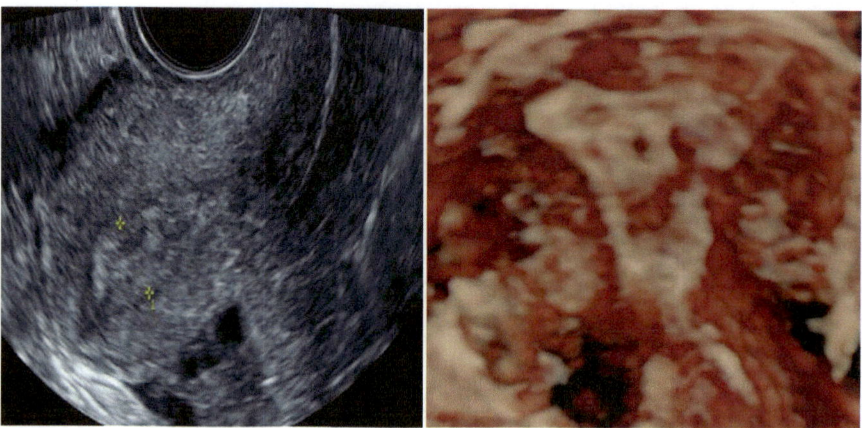

Fig. 6.13 Any inhomogeneity seen in an endometrium on 2D scans (**a**) must be evaluated by 3D to assess for IUAs. In this patient, there is a subtle inhomogeneity. A 3D study (**b**) reveals extensive IUAs superior to the cervix, thick mid and upper cavity adhesions, and bilateral ostial amputation

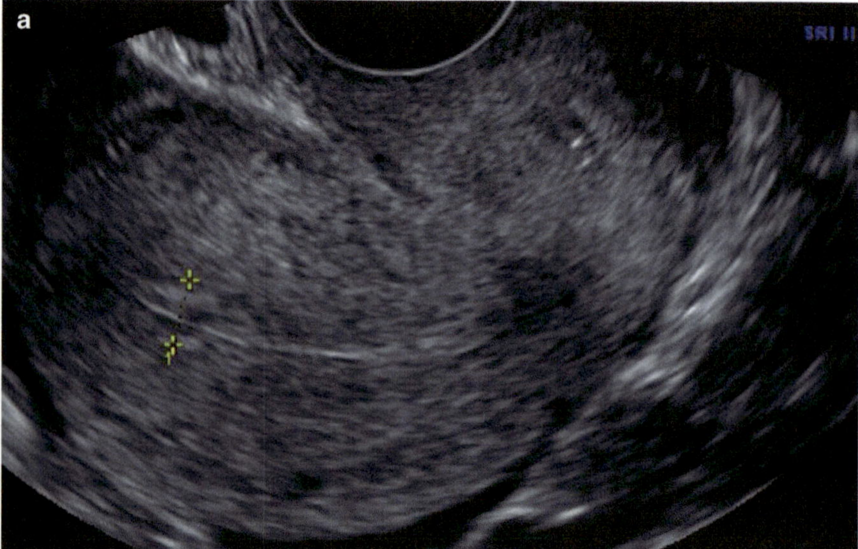

Fig. 6.14 (**a**) Shows a thin, interrupted endometrium that remains as the best ultrasound marker for IUAs. (**b**) Shows 3D rendering using older rendering software that reveals extensive, subtle interruptions. (**c**) Shows newer rendering software that reveals the interruption of the endometrial-myometrial interface with greater diagnostic confidence. (**d**) A multislice display shows extensive obliteration.

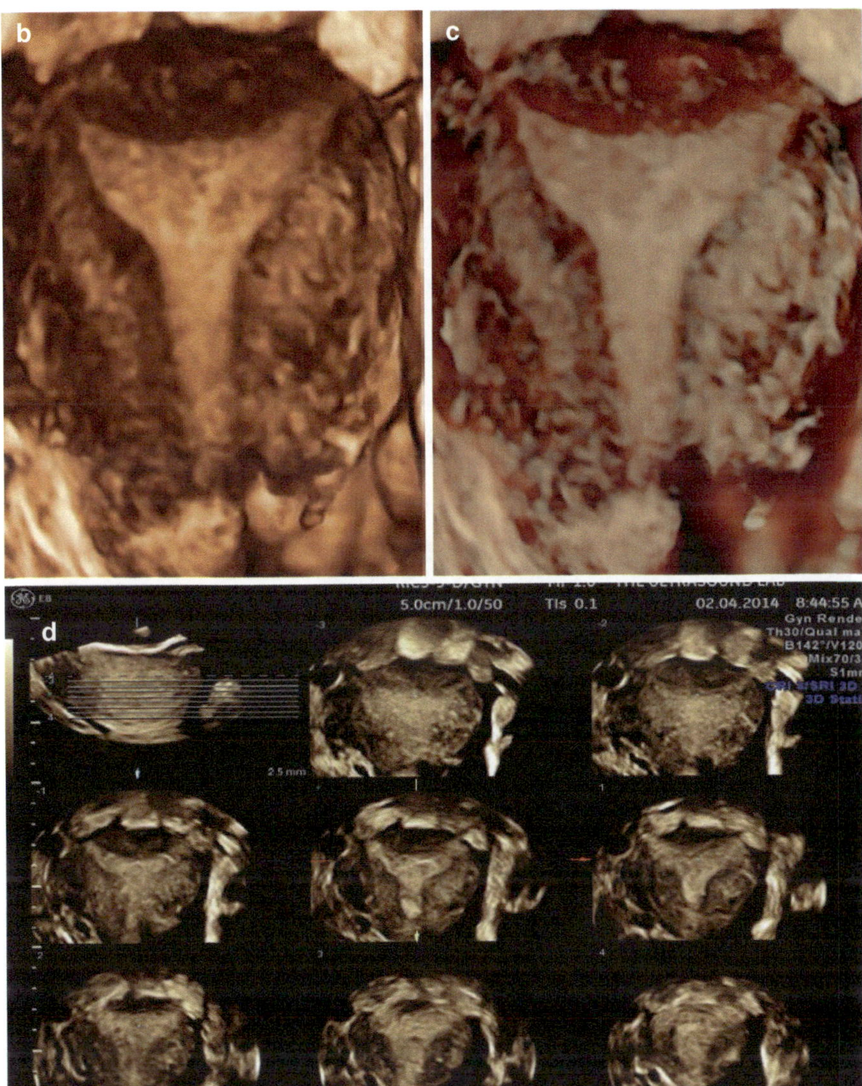

Fig. 6.14 (continued)

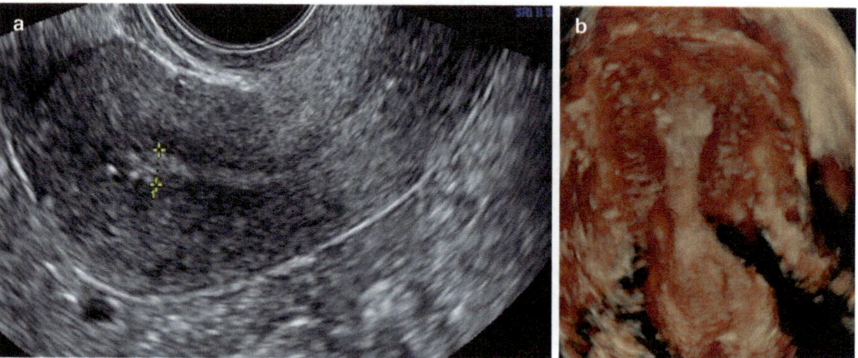

Fig. 6.15 (**a**) Shows endometrial and subendometrial calcifications that are very good markers for the possibility of IUAs in populations with a high incidence of tuberculosis. The true extent of obliteration of the cavity is rarely evident on 2D ultrasound. Figure (**b**) are remarkable at revealing the extent of the disease

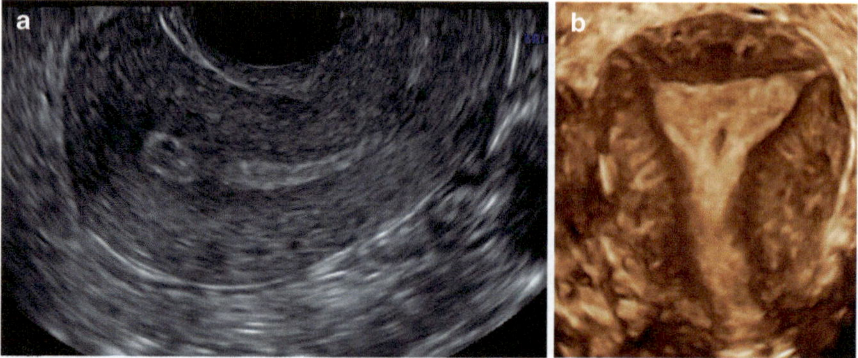

Fig. 6.16 (**a**) 2D studies may reveal large focal interruptions of the cavity. (**b**) Shows 3D studies; it must be added to the evaluation not to confirm the finding, but to assess the lateral margins of the cavity and the morphology of the interstitial course of the tubes

Key Points

1. An optimal diagnostic test should be noninvasive, safe, painless, inexpensive, and applicable to all patients, regardless of their pretest probability of having a particular condition of interest. Ultrasound is the only test that satisfies these criteria.
2. All women should be offered a 3D examination, with or without contrast, in addition to a preliminary 2D transvaginal evaluation.
3. 3D evaluation provides patients and clinicians with self-explanatory images that show the location and extent of cavity obliteration and obstruction. Obliteration should be described subjectively as focal, partial, or complete.

4. Ultrasound has the potential to improve both the safety and efficacy of this procedure by providing preoperative and intraoperative guidance, and postoperative and long-term reevaluation.
5. This has the potential to decrease risks associated with repeated surgery and make the process cost effective.

References

1. Fritsch H. Ein Fall von volligem Schwundser Gebarmutterhohlenach Auskratzung. Zentralbl Gynaekol. 1894;18:1337–42.
2. Asherman JG. Amenorrhoeatraumatica (atretica). J Obstet Gynaecol Br Emp. 1948;55:23–30.
3. Asherman JG. Traumatic intra-uterine adhesions. J Obstet Gynaecol Br Emp. 1950;57:892–6.
4. Yu D, Wong YM, Cheong Y, Xia E, Li TC. Asherman syndrome - one century later. Fertil Steril. 2008;89:759–79.
5. Schenker JG, Margalioth EJ. Intrauterine adhesions: an updated appraisal. Fertil Steril. 1982;37:593–610.
6. Al-Inany H. Intrauterine adhesions: an update. Acta Obstet Gynecol Scand. 2001;80:986–93.
7. Valle RF, Sciarra JJ. Intrauterine adhesions: hysteroscopic diagnosis, classification, treatment, and reproductive outcome. Am J Obstet Gynecol. 1988;158:1459–70.
8. Hooker AB, Lemmers M, Thurkow AL, Heymans MW, Opmeer BC, Brolmann HAM, Mol BW, Huirne JAF. Systematic review and meta-analysis of intrauterine adhesions after miscarriage: prevalence, risk factors and long-term reproductive outcome. Hum Reprod Update. 2014;20:262–78.
9. Xiao S, Wan Y, Xue M, Zeng X, Xiao F, Xu D, Yang X, Zhang P, Sheng W, Xu J, Zhou S. Etiology, treatment, and reproductive prognosis of women with moderate-to-severe intrauterine adhesions. Int J Gynaecol Obstet. 2014;125:121–4.
10. Naftalin J, Jurkovic D. The endometrial–myometrial junction: a fresh look at a busy crossing. Ultrasound Obstet Gynecol. 2009;34:1–11.
11. Amin TN, Saridogan E, Jurkovic D. Ultrasound and intrauterine adhesions: a novel structured approach to diagnosis and management. Ultrasound Obstet Gynecol. 2015;46:131–9.
12. March CM. Intrauterine adhesions. Obstet Gynecol Clin N Am. 1995;22:491–505.
13. Sharma JB, Roy KK, Pushparaj M, Gupta N, Jain SK, Malhotra N, Mittal S. Genital tuberculosis: an important cause of Asherman's syndrome in India. Arch Gynecol Obstet. 2008;277:37–41.
14. Khurana A, Sahi G. Ultrasound in female genital tuberculosis: a retrospective series. Ultrasound Obstet Gynecol. 2013;42:28.
15. Leone FP, Timmerman D, Bourne T, Valentin L, Epstein E, Goldstein SR, Marret H, Parsons AK, Gull B, Istre O, Sepulveda W, Ferrazzi E, Van den Bosch T. Terms, definitions and measurements to describe the sonographic features of the endometrium and intrauterine lesions: a consensus opinion from the International Endometrial Tumor Analysis (IETA) group. Ultrasound Obstet Gynecol. 2010;35:103–12.
16. Wamsteker K, De Blok SJ. Diagnostic hysteroscopy: technique and documentation. In: Sutton C, Diamon M, editors. Endoscopic surgery for gynecologists. New York: Lippincott Williams & Wilkins Publishers; 1995. p. 263–76.
17. The American Fertility Society. Classifications of adnexal adhesions, distal tubal occlusion, tubal occlusion secondary to tubal ligation, tubal pregnancies, mullerian anomalies and intrauterine adhesions. Fertil Steril. 1988;49:944–55.
18. Donnez J, Nisolle M. Hysteroscopic lysis of intrauterine adhesions (Asherman syndrome). In: Donnez J, editor. Atlas of laser operative laparoscopy and hysteroscopy. New York: Press-Parthenon; 1994. p. 305–22.

19. Nasr AL, Al-Inany H, Thabet S, Aboulghar M. A clinicohysteroscopic scoring system of intrauterine adhesions. Gynecol Obstet Investig. 2000;50:178–81.
20. Jones WE. Traumatic intrauterine adhesions. A report of 8 cases with emphasis on therapy. Am J Obstet Gynecol. 1964;89:304–13.
21. Netter AP, Musset R, Lambert A, Salomon Y. Traumatic uterine synechiae: a common cause of menstrual insufficiency, sterility, and abortion. Am J Obstet Gynecol. 1956;71:368–75.
22. Magos A. Hysteroscopic treatment of Asherman's syndrome. Reprod BioMed Online. 2002;4(suppl 3):46–51.
23. Kresowik JD, Syrop CH, Van Voorhis BJ, Ryan GL. Ultrasound is the optimal choice for guidance in difficult hysteroscopy. Ultrasound Obstet Gynecol. 2012;39:715–8.
24. Tan IF, Robertson M. The role of imaging in the investigation of Asherman's syndrome. AJUM. 2011;14:15–8.
25. Roma Dalfo A, Ubeda B, Ubeda A, Monzon M, Rotger R, Ramos R, Palacio A. Diagnostic value of hysterosalpingography in the detection of intrauterine abnormalities: a comparison with hysteroscopy. AJR Am J Roentgenol. 2004;183:1405–9.
26. Soares SR, Barbosa dos Reis MM, Camargos AF. Diagnostic accuracy of sonohysterography, transvaginal sonography, and hysterosalpingography in patients with uterine cavity diseases. Fertil Steril. 2000;73:406–11.
27. Raziel A, Arieli S, Bukovsky I, Caspi E, Golan A. Investigation of the uterine cavity in recurrent aborters. Fertil Steril. 1994;62:1080–2.
28. Fayez JA, Mutie G, Schneider PJ. The diagnostic value of hysterosalpingography and hysteroscopy in infertility investigation. Am J Obstet Gynecol. 1987;156:558–60.
29. Salle B, Gaucherand P, de Saint HP, Rudigoz RC. Transvaginal sonohysterographic evaluation of intrauterine adhesions. J Clin Ultrasound. 1999;27:131–4.
30. Sylvestre C, Child TJ, Tulandi T, Tan SL. A prospective study to evaluate the efficacy of two- and three-dimensional sonohysterography in women with intrauterine lesions. Fertil Steril. 2003;79:1222–5.
31. Laganà AS, Ciancimino L, Mancuso A, Chiofalo B, Rizzo P, Triolo O. 3D sonohysterography vs hysteroscopy: a cross-sectional study for the evaluation of endouterine diseases. Arch Gynecol Obstet. 2014;290:1173–8.
32. Malhotra N, Bahadur A, Kalaivani M, Mittal S. Changes in endometrial receptivity in women with Asherman's syndrome undergoing hysteroscopic adhesiolysis. Arch Gynecol Obstet. 2012;286:525–30.
33. Ludwin A, Ludwin I, Kudla M, Pitynski K, Banas T, Jach R, Knafel A. Diagnostic accuracy of three-dimensional sonohysterography compared with office hysteroscopy and its interrater/intrarater agreement in uterine cavity assessment after hysteroscopic metroplasty. Fertil Steril. 2014;101:1392–9.
34. Cullinan JA, Fleischer AC, Kepple DM, Arnold AL. Sonohysterography: a technique for endometrial evaluation. Radiographics. 1995;15:501–14; discussion 515–516.
35. Parsons AK, Lense JJ. Sonohysterography for endometrial abnormalities: preliminary results. J Clin Ultrasound. 1993;21:87–95.
36. Yan L, Wang A, Bai R, Shang W, Zhao Y, Wang W, Guo W. Application of Sono Vue combined with three-dimensional color power angiography in the diagnosis and prognosis evaluation of intrauterine adhesion. Eur J Obstet Gynecol Reprod Biol. 2016;198:68–72.
37. Fedele L, Bianchi S, Dorta M, Vignali M. Intrauterine adhesions: detection with transvaginal US. Radiology. 1996;199:757–9.
38. AAGL Elevating Gynecologic Surgery Gynecological Surgery. AAGL practice report: practice guidelines on intrauterine adhesions developed in collaboration with the European Society of Gynaecological Endoscopy (ESGE). Gynecol Surg. 2017;14(1):6.
39. Knopman J, Copperman AB. Value of 3D ultrasound in the management of suspected Asherman's syndrome. J Reprod Med. 2007;52:1016–22.
40. Salim R, Lee C, Davies A, Jolaoso B, Ofuasia E, Jurkovic D. A comparative study of three-dimensional saline infusion sonohysterography and diagnostic hysteroscopy for the classification of submucous fibroids. Hum Reprod. 2005;20:253–7.

41. Jurkovic D. Three-dimensional ultrasound in gynecology: a critical evaluation. Ultrasound Obstet Gynecol. 2002;19:109–17.
42. Bacelar AC, Wilcock D, Powell M, Worthington BS. The value of MRI in the assessment of traumatic intra-uterine adhesions (Asherman's syndrome). Clin Radiol. 1995;50:80–3.
43. Dykes TA, Isler RJ, McLean AC. MR imaging of Asherman syndrome: total endometrial obliteration. J Comput Assist Tomogr. 1991;15:858–60.
44. Letterie GS, Haggerty MF. Magnetic resonance imaging of intrauterine synechiae. Gynecol Obstet Investig. 1994;37:66–8.
45. Takeuchi M, Matsuzaki K, Nishitani H. Diffusion-weighted magnetic resonance imaging of endometrial cancer: differentiation from benign endometrial lesions and preoperative assessment of myometrial invasion. Acta Radiol. 2009;50:947–53.

Role of Hysterosalpingography (HSG) and Sono-HSG

7

Nitin P. Ghonge, Sanchita Dube Ghonge, and Alka Ashmita Singhal

7.1 Introduction

Hysterosalpingography (HSG) has become an important initial investigation in patients who present with infertility or other endometrial/tubal problems. This chapter predominantly deals with HSG as the initial screening procedure for an intrauterine adhesion or Asherman's workup with emphasis on procedural details and image interpretation. It also briefly addresses the ultrasound extension of HSG–sono-HSG and its advantages over HSG.

7.2 Hysterosalpingography (HSG)

This is the radiographic imaging of uterine cavity, fallopian tubes, peritoneal cavity, and cervical canal, during intracavitary injection of contrast media under fluoroscopic visualization. Though the procedure is in practice for more than 100 years now, HSG is now increasingly being performed [1]. This is likely to be due to increase in the number of patients presenting with the problem of infertility as well as the recent advances in the field of reproductive medicine. Hysterosalpingography is considered an initial screening procedure for an infertility workup, and despite the development of other diagnostic tools including MRI, hysteroscopy, and laparoscopy, HSG remains the main examination for the study of the fallopian tubes [2].

N. P. Ghonge (✉)
Department of Radiology, Indraprastha Apollo Hospitals, New Delhi, India

S. D. Ghonge
Department of Obstetrics and Gynecology, Apollo Hospital, Noida, India

A. A. Singhal
Medanta Division of Radiology and Nuclear Medicine, Medanta the Medicity Hospital, Delhi, India

R. Manchanda (ed.), *Intra Uterine Adhesions*,
https://doi.org/10.1007/978-981-33-4145-6_7

In general, ultrasound is considered to be more effective for endometrial imaging: MRI for myometrial imaging and HSG for tubal imaging. In infertility workup, HSG has been reported to have high sensitivity but low specificity, particularly in the evaluation of endometrial abnormalities [3]. The technical quality of HSG and the image interpretation skills play an important role in the performance of HSG in these patients [4]. The concerns about the technical and interpretation lapses in HSG were highlighted in a questionnaire-based study [5]. The study included 50 radiologists and 50 gynecologists, irrespective of their practice settings and years of experience. The study revealed few serious lapses in the procedure and interpretation of HSG which can account for the inferior diagnostic performance and can certainly be improved with awareness, education, and training.

Hysteroscopy is the gold standard of methods for diagnosis of intrauterine adhesions, against which all others must be compared. Hysterosalpingography (HSG) is a useful screening outpatient radiological procedure for diagnosis and has 75% sensitivity, 95% specificity, 50% positive predictive value (PPV), and 98% negative predictive value (NPV). Considerable interobserver variability in the interpretation of HSGs has been reported, depending on the type of pathology being assessed. Women with possible comorbidity such as pelvic and tubal diseases may need a laparoscopic assessment.

For greatest accuracy, it is important to perform HSG without a speculum in the vagina and, if a balloon catheter is used, to deflate the balloon before ending the examination to ensure that the entire cavity has been adequately visualized. Mild-to-moderate intrauterine adhesions generally yield irregular filling defects in a lacunar pattern and may be identified in any region of the uterine cavity.

When adhesions are severe, it may be impossible to visualize the endometrial cavity altogether. The fluoroscopic exposure (radiation exposure) associated with a normal HSG is approximately 63 s (range 17–404 s) when the test is normal and 100 s (range 28–172 s) when abnormal.

Mild-to-moderate cramping pain is commonly associated with HSG and can be minimized by treatment with nonsteroidal anti-inflammatory agents beginning approximately 1 h before the procedure. Pelvic infections, vagal reactions, intravasation of contrast, and iodine-induced allergic reactions are uncommon but potentially serious complications of HSG.

7.3 Patient Selection

7.3.1 Indications and Contraindications

Apart from the IUA workup, HSG may be advised for a wide range of clinical indications. Based on the clinical settings, appropriate patient selection is important for performing the HSG. The other clinical indications and contraindications for HSG are mentioned in Fig. 7.1 [6].

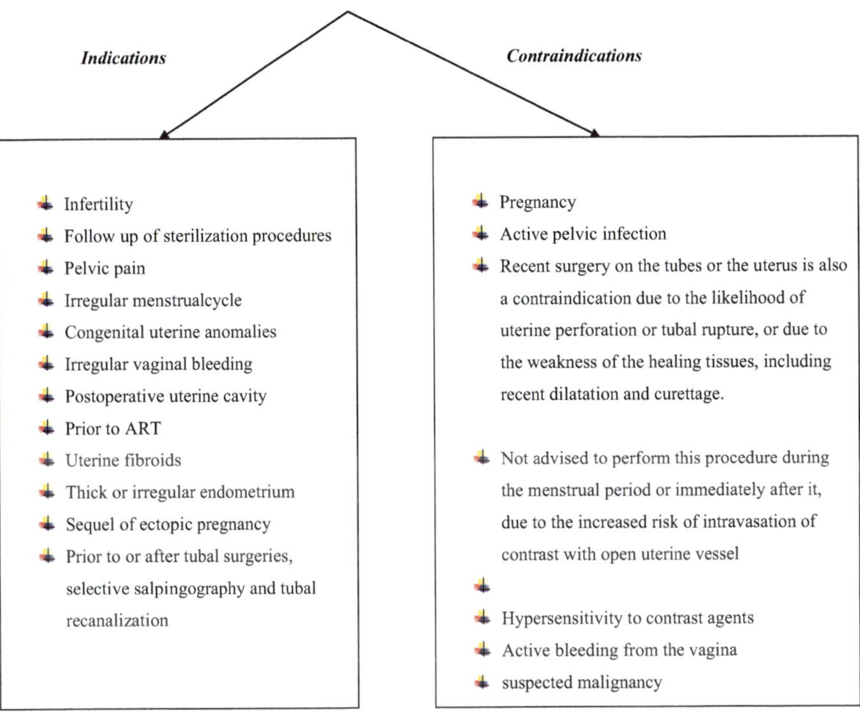

Fig. 7.1 Patient selection

7.3.2 Preparation

- As pregnancy is the absolute contraindication, 10-day rule should be followed.
- HSG should be scheduled during the follicular phase of the menstrual cycle, after menstrual flow has ceased but before the patient has ovulated, usually between 7th and 10th days of menstrual cycle. HSG before the 7th day may increase the chances of contrast intravasation into the fragile veins and therefore adversely affect the image interpretation.
- The patient should be instructed to abstain from sexual intercourse from the time menstrual bleeding ends until the day of the study to avoid a potential pregnancy.
- If the patient has irregular menstrual cycles or there is a possibility of pregnancy, serum beta HCG level should be evaluated.
- HSG should not be performed when ongoing pelvic infection or active vaginal bleeding is present.
- Patients with cervical stenosis may pose difficulty due to difficulty in cervical cannulation and may be initially treated.
- History of allergy or idiosyncratic reaction to iodinated contrast media is a relative contraindication and may require premedication with diphenhydramine, steroids, and/or other medications.

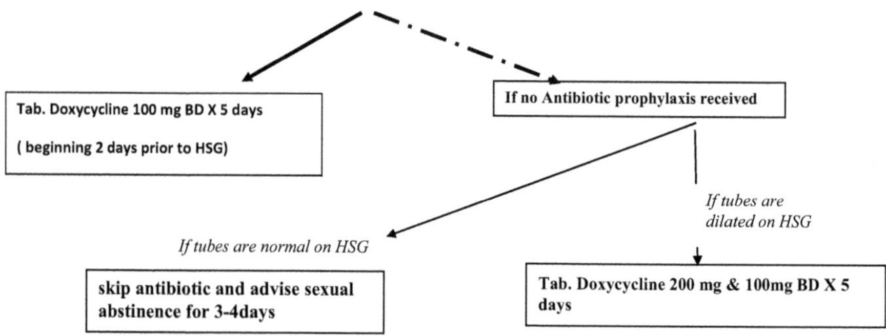

Fig. 7.2 Antibiotic prophylaxis for HSG

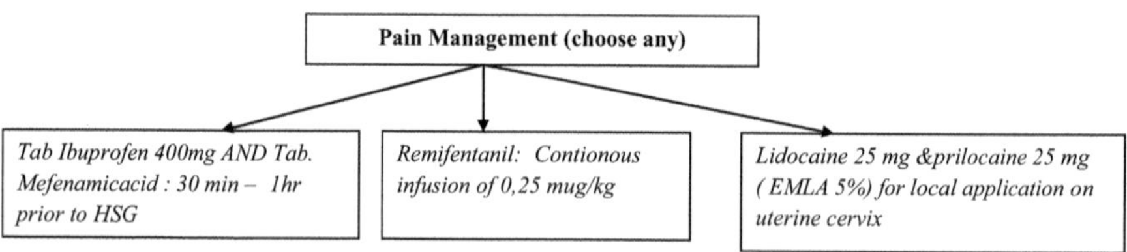

Fig. 7.3 Pain management (choose any)

- Though pre-procedural antibiotics are not advised in all the patients, it should be considered in patients with a history of pelvic inflammatory disease or with cardiac lesions.
- A practical recommendation for the use of antibiotics is stated in Fig. 7.2 [7]. Antibiotics may also be advised in patients after hydrosalpinx is diagnosed on HSG.
- Pre-procedural analgesia is important to ensure painless patient experience and to avoid the vasovagal response during the procedure. The clinical practice often varies across different institutions. List of different drug combinations is stated in Fig. 7.3 [8, 9].

7.3.3 Procedural Technique

The patient is asked to empty her bladder and then lie supine on the fluoroscopy table in the lithotomy position.

The perineum is prepared with povidone-iodine solution and draped with sterile towels.

A speculum is inserted into the vagina. The cervix is localized and cleansed with povidone-iodine solution.

Metal or plastic Leech Wilkinson HSG cannula is used depending upon the institute's practice (Fig. 7.4).

During traditional HSG, a vulsellum or tenaculum is placed on the anterior cervical lip of the external cervical os for traction. It is placed at 12 o'clock position as cervical vascularity is greatest at 3 o'clock and 9 o'clock positions, and therefore avoided. There are many catheter systems including rigid systems or flexible catheters with and without a balloon system [7]. Patients with a patulous or incompetent cervix are best examined with the 5F balloon systems or an 8-French pediatric Foley catheter. The balloon should be filled with fluid to avoid artifact. Balloon catheters usually do not require tenaculum placement for cervical traction.

The cannula is placed just beyond the internal os. Several modifications in technique may be required. External compression over the pubic symphysis is likely to bring the cervix into view in patients with posterior location of cervix (Fig. 7.5).

Valsalva maneuver is useful to improve cervical visualization particularly in multiparous or grand multiparous patients.

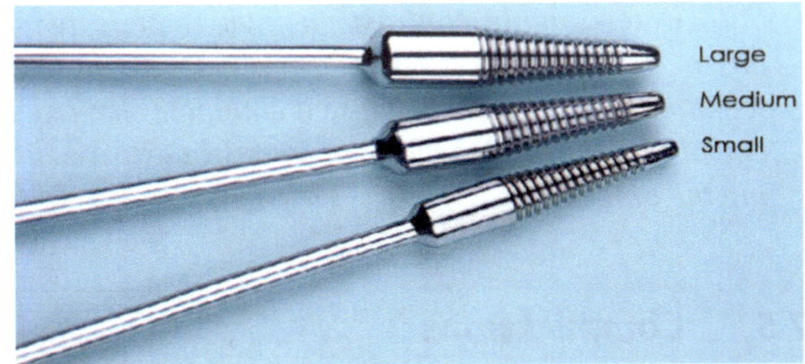

Fig. 7.4 Leech Wilkinson cannula

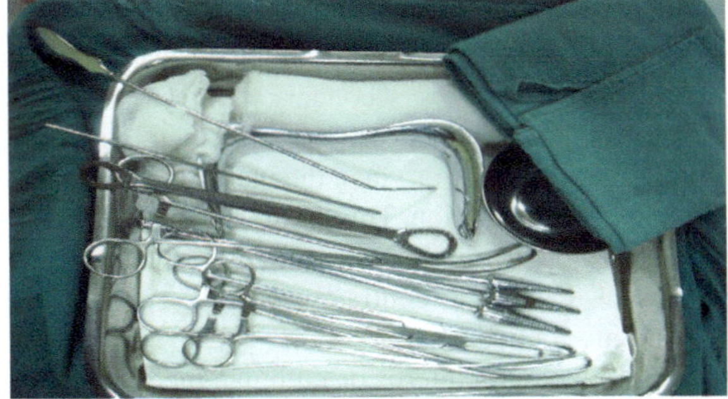

Fig. 7.5 Instruments required for HSG (Sims speculum, anterior vaginal wall retractor, uterine sound, vulsellum, Allis forceps, HSG cannula)

7.4 Radiological Contrast Used in HSG

The choice of contrast material for HSG is often debated as few authors support the use of an oil-soluble contrast medium, as this is likely to provide greater contrast and image sharpness and better evaluate peri-tubal adhesions [10].

An increase in pregnancy rates in infertile patients after HSG with oil-soluble medium has been suggested [11] whereas another study [12] shows no statistical difference between the use of oil- and water-soluble contrast agents.

A recent multicenter [13], randomized trial in 27 hospitals in the Netherlands randomly assigned the patients with infertility into oil-based contrast or water-based contrast groups. A total of 220 of 554 women in the oil-based group (39.7%) and 161 of 554 women in the water-based group (29.1%) conceived (rate ratio 1.37; 95% confidence interval [CI] 1.16 to 1.61; $P < 0.001$), and 214 of 552 women in the oil-based group (38.8%) and 155 of 552 women in the water-based group (28.1%) had live births (rate ratio 1.38; 95% CI 1.17 to 1.64; $P < 0.001$). Rates of pregnancy and live births were significantly higher among women who underwent HSG with oil-based contrast as compared to women who had HSG with water-based contrast in this study.

- *Still, water-soluble contrast medium is preferred at most institutions due to absence of any serious secondary effects like peritoneal inflammatory or granulomatous reaction and because it eliminates the risk of pulmonary and retinal oil emboli during the inadvertent venous in extravasation of contrast medium during the procedure.*

7.5 Complications

- Bleeding and infection are the most common complications of HSG. The patient should be made aware about the possibility of light spotting after the procedure, usually lasting less than 24 h.
- Mild fever or foul-smelling vaginal discharge over the 2–4-day period following the procedure may be secondary to infection.
- Patients may experience cramping when the catheter balloon is inflated in the endocervical canal or when the uterus is overdistended with contrast material or with tubal obstruction. This cramping is generally minor and transient and is well tolerated by the majority of patients.
- Risk of reaction to contrast material is very low with the use of low-osmolar nonionic contrast agents.
- Perforation of the uterus or fallopian tubes is extremely unlikely with the use of optimal technique.
- Appropriate timing of the examination and a negative pregnancy test should minimize the possible chances of irradiation of an unsuspected pregnancy.

7.6 Image Acquisition

Plain radiograph of the pelvis is obtained with the catheter in place before contrast material is instilled with the side marker in place. Water-soluble iodinated contrast (ionic or nonionic) is slowly injected under fluoroscopy guidance.

7.6.1 Standard Set of Images (Fig. 7.6a–d) Include

FIRST IMAGE obtained during early filling of the uterus to evaluate for any focal/ linear filling defect due to polyp/mass lesion or adhesion in the endometrial cavity. Small subtle filling defects are best seen at this stage.

SECOND IMAGE is obtained with the uterus fully distended to evaluate the uterine contour. The fallopian tubes are also optimally opacified and delineated in this image for course and caliber.

THIRD IMAGE is expected to delineate the free or loculated intraperitoneal spillage of the contrast to assess tubal patency.

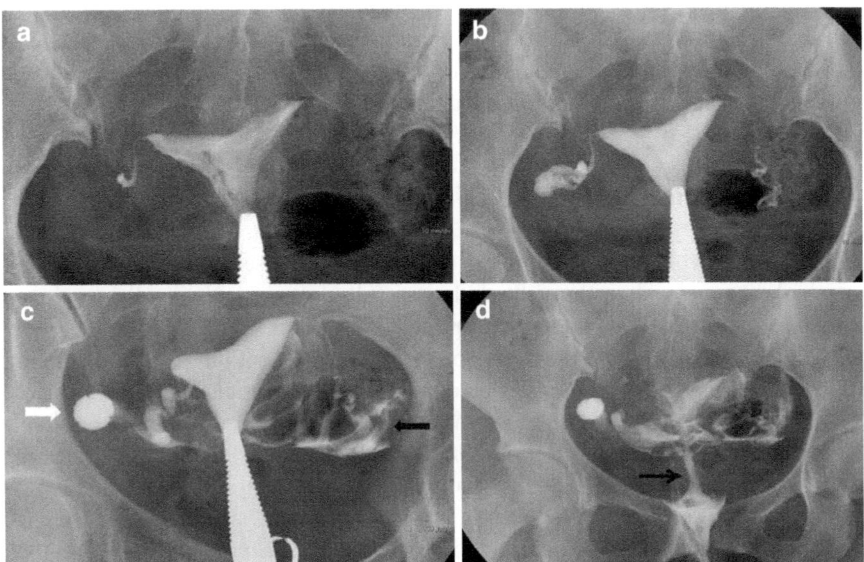

Fig. 7.6 (**a–d**) Standard set of images to be acquired during HSG. (**a**) Shows early endometrial filling to look for small lesions, (**b**) endometrial cavity for uterine shape and contour, (**c**) white arrow showing right-sided hydrosalpinx without spillage and black arrow showing normal spillage, (**d**) post-cannula removal film for evaluation of uterine cervix (thin black arrow). Slow and steady contrast injection is necessary to ensure image acquisition in different phases

FOURTH IMAGE is acquired soon after the removal of metal or plastic cannula to delineate the endocervical canal for focal filling defects. It is important to ensure that the contrast injection rate is slow and uniform to ensure acquisition of images in different phases. Additional images including pelvic inlet views, oblique views, or delayed spot views may be acquired in selective cases depending upon the findings.

Just before removing the cannula, "pull-release" maneuver may be performed to assess the degree of pelvic peritoneal adhesions. Apart from this, extravasated contrast is likely to track along the external uterine fundal surface following the maneuver, which provides vital clues in the evaluation of uterine mullerian anomaly.

7.6.2 Equipment Specifications

HSG must always be performed with fluoroscopic equipment meeting all applicable federal, state, and local radiation standards [6]. The equipment should provide diagnostic fluoroscopic image quality and recording capability. The equipment should be capable of producing kilovoltage greater than 100 kVp. Fluoroscopy equipment with the ability to hold the last image is necessary. Appropriate emergency equipment and medications must be immediately available to treat adverse reactions associated with administered medications. The equipment and medications should be monitored for inventory and drug expiration dates on a regular basis. The equipment, medications, and other emergency support must also be appropriate for the range of ages and sizes in the patient population.

7.7 Radiation Dosage and Safety

As the HSG involves use of ionizing radiation, patient selection is an important step and diagnostic algorithms should be carefully followed. Nationally developed guidelines, such as the ACR's Appropriateness Criteria, should be used to help choose the most appropriate imaging procedures to prevent unwarranted radiation exposure. If justified, HSG should be done with the minimum radiation exposure necessary to provide sufficient anatomic detail for diagnosis of normal or abnormal findings. Adherence to the appropriate practice parameters will maximize the diagnostic benefit of HSG and ensure optimal patient safety. Risk-benefit analysis should be performed for each case.

Radiation hygiene is an important component of HSG procedure and ALARA [as low as reasonably achievable] principles should be followed. Accordingly, due care must be taken to minimize the radiation dose without compromising the quality. To achieve this objective use of digital fluoroscopy is better for HSG, as there is precise control over the radiation dose. Intermittent fluoroscopy should be performed during the procedure. With mean fluoroscopy time of 0.3 min, the average gonad dose is approximately 270 cGy and the effective dose is 1.2 mSv [14].

Radiologists, medical physicists, registered radiologist assistants, radiologic technologists, and all supervising physicians have a responsibility for radiation safety in the workplace by keeping radiation exposure to patients, staff, and society as a whole, "as low as reasonably achievable" (ALARA). Automated dose reduction technologies available on imaging equipment should be used whenever appropriate. Otherwise, appropriate manual techniques should be used.

Additional information regarding patient radiation safety is available at the Image Wisely websites [15]. "Image Wisely" is a joint initiative of the American College of Radiology, Radiological Society of North America, American Society of Radiological Technologists, and American Association of Physicists in Medicine. These global awareness campaigns provide free educational materials for all the patients, technologists, referring clinicians, medical physicists, and radiologists. Radiation exposures should be measured and regular auditing should be performed by a qualified medical physicist in accordance with the applicable technical standards and guidelines [16].

7.8 Normal Appearances and Imaging Pitfalls in HSG

On HSG, the uterus should be seen as an inverted triangle with well-defined, smooth contours (Fig. 7.7a). Anteverted or retroverted uterine position may have significant impact on the appearance of normal uterus. Similarly, the rotation of uterus along the long axis may not show the profile views of the uterine cornu. The anteroinferior traction on the uterine cervix is likely to straighten the uterus and minimize the impact of position or rotation of the uterus. The uterus should be evaluated for abnormal filling defects due to focal lesion in the endometrial cavity or for the altered shape and position secondary to uterine mullerian anomaly or due to presence of space-occupying lesion in the endometrial cavity, myometrium, or pelvis.

It is important to be cautious of linear filling defects along the long axis of uterus in the early filling defects due to mucosal folds and it should not be assumed to be pathological (Fig. 7.7b).

Care should be taken to flush the catheter thoroughly with contrast material to avoid injecting air bubbles. Air bubbles manifest as well-circumscribed rounded filling defects in the nondependent portion of the uterus (Fig. 7.7c). They are often mobile and transient and should always be differentiated from fixed filling defects. Cesarean section scars may be seen as focal outpouching or irregularity at the typical location in the lower uterine segment in the region of the isthmus.

The cervical canal is opacified during HSG and shows varied appearance depending upon the parity of the patient. The cervical canal is usually narrower at external and internal os and wider in the midportion. The walls may be smooth or serrated with longitudinal ridges. Prominent serrated appearance (plicae palmatae) is often more prominently seen in nulliparous females (Fig. 7.7d).

Venous or lymphatic intravasation may occur during HSG, which may interfere with optimal image interpretation. Though it may occur in healthy patients, few predisposing factors include recent uterine surgery or instrumentation, increased

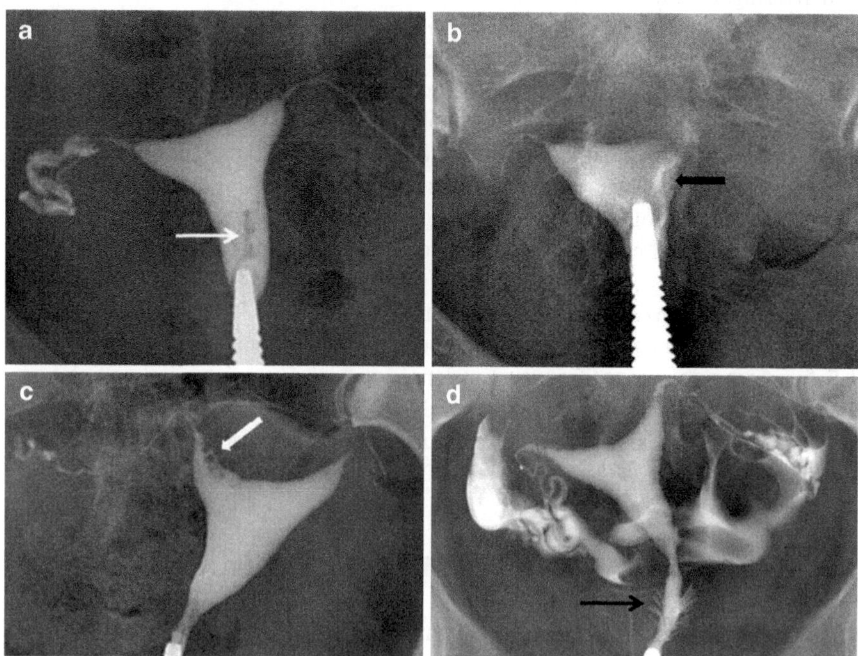

Fig. 7.7 (**a–d**) Normal appearance and pitfalls. Uterus should be seen as an inverted triangle with well-defined, smooth contour on HSG (**a**). Dislodged mucous plug is at times seen as linear filling defect (white thin arrow). Linear filling defects may be seen along the long axis of uterus in the early filling defects due to mucosal folds (**b**, black thick arrow). Air bubbles may be seen as well-circumscribed rounded filling defects (**c**, white thick arrow). Prominent serrated appearance (plicae palmatae) is often seen in nulliparous females (**d**, black thin arrow)

intrauterine pressure because of tubal obstruction, or excessive pressure during the injection. The radiographic appearance of early intravasation is characterized by filling of multiple thin tortuous beaded channels with vertical or oblique course with or without delineation of the ovarian vein (Fig. 7.8).

The normal appearances of fallopian tubes on HSG should be clearly understood. The fallopian tubes measure approximately 10 cm and are seen as linear tubular structures on both sides which show varied appearances and caliber in different parts (Fig. 7.9a). From medial to lateral ends, the medial most part is the interstitial or cornual segment, which extends from the uterine cavity through the uterine muscle and continues into the isthmic segment. The interstitial and isthmic segments are often divided by a thin linear filling defect on HSG. The isthmus is the narrow muscular portion adjacent to the uterus, which is seen as linear/curvilinear thin structure. The isthmus gradually continues as the ampullary segment which is wider and longer middle part of the tube. Characteristically, this part shows longitudinal linear filling defects due to presence of prominent mucosal folds (Fig. 7.9b). Ampulla terminates into infundibular segment laterally which is a funnel-shaped segment next to the fimbrial end. The infundibulum segment and

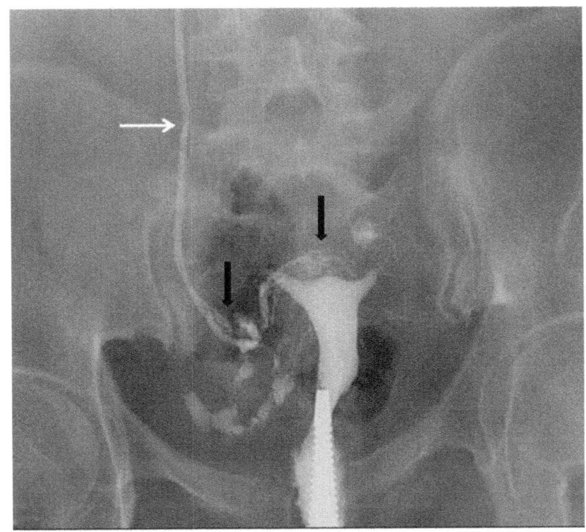

Fig. 7.8 HSG image showing early intravasation into myometrial and para-tubal veins (black arrows). Venous intravasation may also lead to opacification and delineation of the ovarian veins (white arrow)

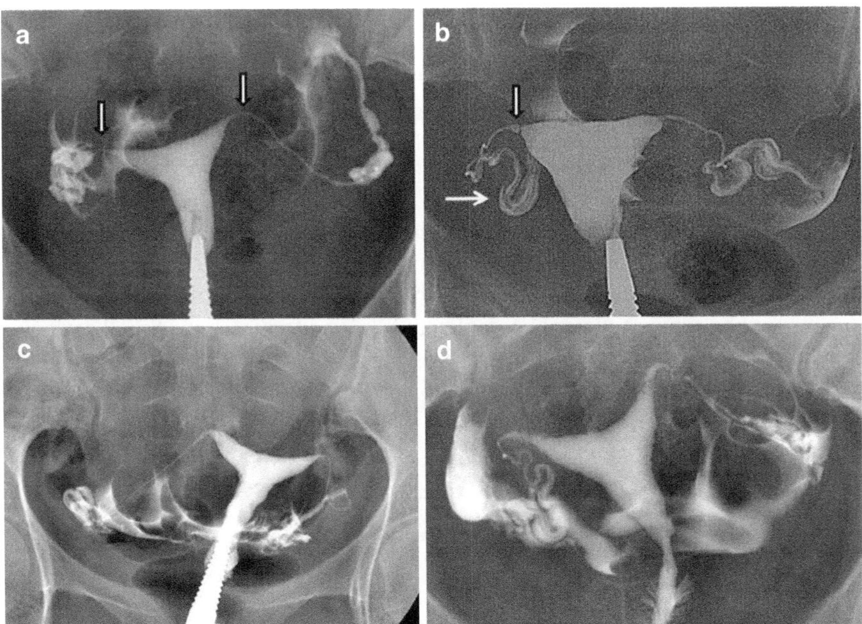

Fig. 7.9 HSG image showing different parts of fallopian tubes on each side (vertical arrows; **a**). The interstitial and isthmic segments are often divided by a thin linear filling defect on HSG at the uterine cornu (vertical arrow; **b**). The isthmus is the narrow muscular portion adjacent to uterus, which is seen as linear/curvilinear thin structure. The isthmus gradually continues as the ampullary segment which is wider and longer middle part of the tube. Characteristically, this part shows longitudinal linear filling defects due to the presence of normal mucosal folds (horizontal arrow, **b**). Free spillage of contrast during HSG should always delineate the peritoneal folds including the region of pouch of Douglas (**c**, **d**)

the fimbrial ends are not seen separately and are only seen as focal flaring of the lateral end of the tube.

The injected contrast during the HSG is expected to show normal spillage into the peritoneal cavity. The spillage of contrast into the peritoneal cavity should be carefully evaluated to decide if it is free spillage of localized spillage. Free spillage should always delineate the peritoneal folds including the region of pouch of Douglas (Fig. 7.9c, d).

7.9 Role of HSG

7.9.1 Presence of Abnormal Endometrial Filling Defects (Fig. 7.10)

Presence of intracavitary filling defect often suggests presence of intra-endometrial lesion.

- **SYNECHIAE** are intrauterine adhesions that result from scarring secondary to the endometrial trauma of curettage procedure or due to endometrial infections.

Early adhesions—Linear or curvilinear filling defects in the endometrial cavity (Fig. 7.11a).

Extensive adhesions—The cavity may show gradually progressive mucosal surface irregularity, altered shape, reduction in the volume, and poor distension of the endometrial cavity (Fig. 7.11b, c).

Endometrial polyps are focal polypoidal areas of hypertrophied endometrium and are seen as well-defined filling defects, more conspicuously during the early filling stage (Fig. 7.12). Small polyps may be obscured in the late distended phase of injection when contrast material completely fills the uterine cavity. Small endometrial polyp and submucosal myoma may not be distinguishable on HSG and would require transvaginal ultrasound examination.

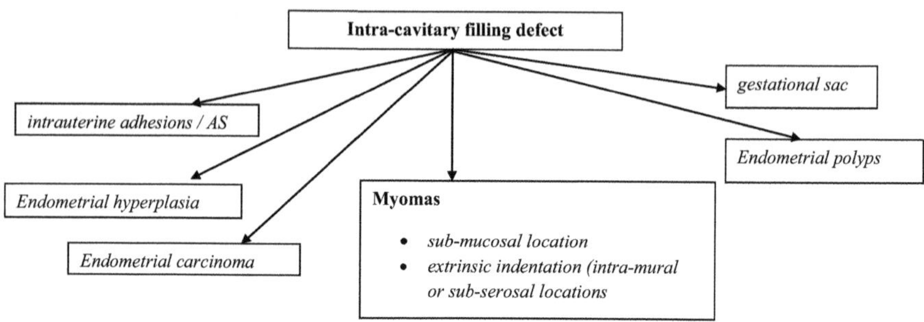

Fig. 7.10 Intracavitary filling defect

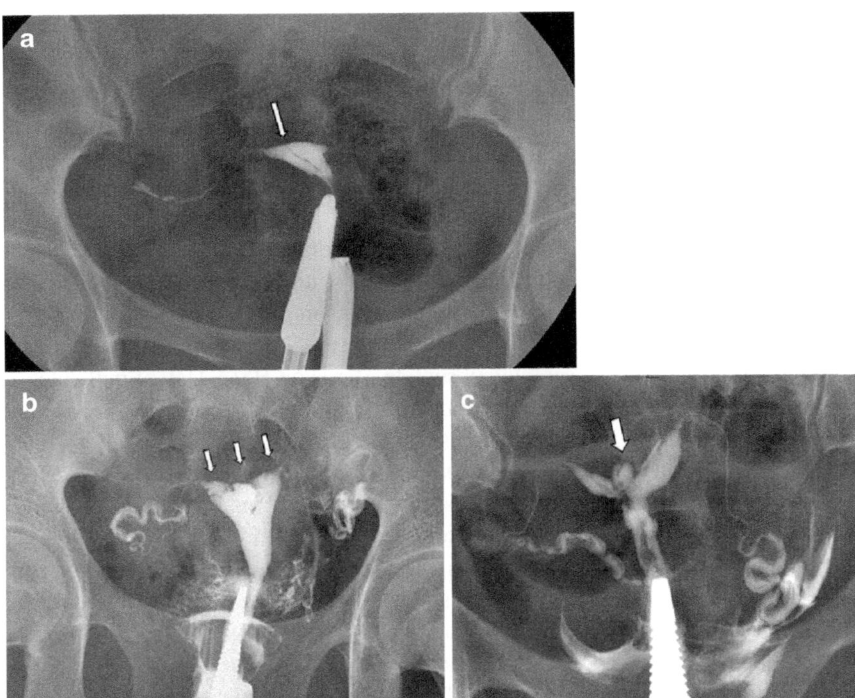

Fig. 7.11 (**a**) HSG image showing the presence of linear filling defect in the endometrial cavity extending up to fundal surface which suggested early endometrial adhesions. (**b**, **c**) Radiographic acquisition in the early filling phase is necessary to detect early changes as illustrated here. With extensive adhesions as in Asherman's syndrome, the cavity may show gradually progressive mucosal surface irregularity, altered shape, reduction in the volume, and poor distension of the endometrial cavity. The endometrial adhesive process may or may not be associated with disease in the fallopian tubes

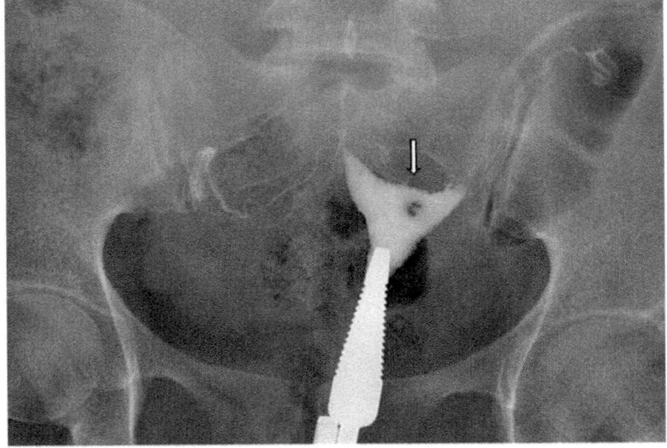

Fig. 7.12 HSG image showing a rounded filling defect in the endometrial cavity secondary to focal endometrial polyp (arrow). Mild surface irregularity is also noted in the endometrial cavity

7.9.2 Altered Uterine Shape and Contour

A detailed evaluation of the uterine shape and contour is an integral component of HSG as it provides vital clues about uterine mullerian anomaly or presence of pelvic space-occupying lesion. The uterine margins should be carefully evaluated with particular emphasis on the fundal region. The shape of the uterus and the status of external fundal surface are important morphological parameters for diagnosis and typing of the uterine mullerian anomaly [17, 18]. Tubular laterally located [banana-shaped] endometrial cavity with presence of single ipsilateral tube is usually seen in unicornuate uterus. Complete or partial duplication of the endometrial cavity is nicely delineated on HSG to diagnose uterine didelphys, bicornuate uterus, or septate/subseptate uterus on HSG. Use of pull-release maneuver is likely to provide important information about the external fundal surface for precise interpretation. The septate/subseptate uterus is likely to have shallow indentation (<10 mm) along the external uterine surface as compared to deep indentation in patients with bicornuate uterus. This important parameter is however better delineated on ultrasound or MRI. Additional morphological parameters which may be evaluated on HSG include intercornual angle and distance. Intercornual angle less than 75° suggests septate uterus while intercornual angle more than 105° suggests bicornuate uterus. Angles measuring 75°–105° are indeterminate in this differentiation. Intercornual distance more than 4 cm usually suggests bicornuate uterus. Presence of broad-based indentation over the fundus with flattening of the external surface with partial duplication of the endometrial cavity is suggestive of arcuate uterus.

Depending upon the size and location, uterine leiomyomas may be seen as either focal filling defect (submucosal location) or extrinsic indentation (intramural or subserosal locations) with or without deformity of the uterine shape (Fig. 7.13).

Sono-HSG is a better imaging option for effective diagnosis, characterization, and exact localization of the uterine intra-endometrial or submucosal lesions.

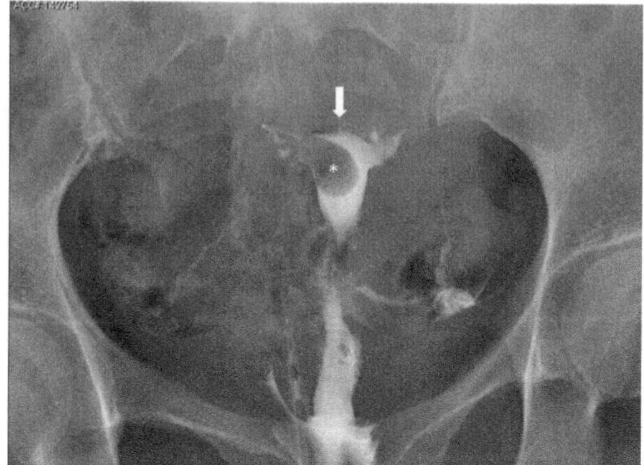

Fig. 7.13 HSG image showing large filling defect (marked as *) in the right pericornual location of uterus [arrow] with non-opacification of the right fallopian tube. Uterine leiomyomas may be seen as either focal filling defect (submucosal location) or extrinsic indentation (intramural or subserosal locations)

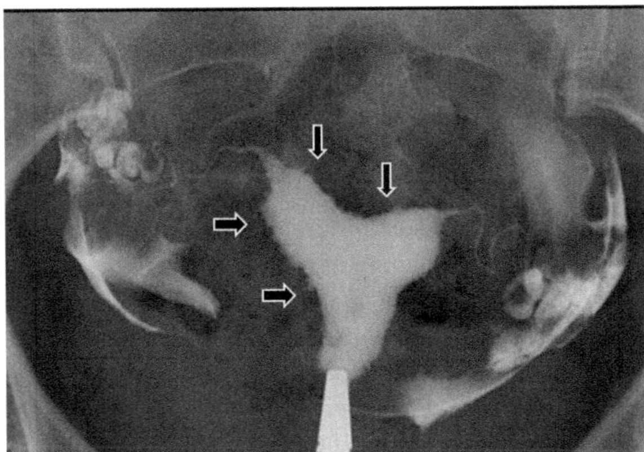

Fig. 7.14 HSG image showing the presence of multiple small diverticula (arrows) along the endometrial cavity extending into the inner myometrium, which is suggestive of uterine adenomyosis. Preserved uterine shape and volume points against the possibility of endometritis or adhesions. Bilateral tubes are patent with preserved course and caliber

Though MRI is the gold standard for imaging diagnosis of adenomyosis, they may be suspected on HSG with the presence of multiple small diverticula extending into the inner myometrium (Fig. 7.14). Inadvertent HSG performed during the ongoing pregnancy may show gestational sac as a focal rounded filling defect on HSG and should be confirmed with prompt ultrasound examination in suspected cases. The procedure should be immediately abandoned and dose calculations performed to decide the continuation or termination of pregnancy.

7.10 Role of HSG in Tubal and Peritoneal Evaluation

Tubal abnormalities seen at HSG may be due to either spasm or secondary to luminal occlusion or infection. The cornual portion of fallopian tube is encased by the smooth muscle of the uterus. If there is spasm of the muscle during HSG, one or both tubes may not fill beyond the corneal portion of the tube. Tubal spasm cannot be distinguished from tubal occlusion on the basis of imaging signs. Administration of spasmolytic agent like glucagon may result in uterine muscle relaxation and help to differentiate tubal spasm from true occlusion [19].

Evaluation of tubal patency is one of the prime objectives of HSG in infertility workup.

Tubal occlusion is seen as abrupt cutoff of intraluminal contrast with non-opacification of distal fallopian tube, which may be unilateral or bilateral and may involve any portion of the tube. If the occlusion is in the ampullary portion, the tube may dilate and form hydrosalpinx. The dilated tubal segments may be focal or segmental. PID is the most common cause of tubal occlusion leading to infertility. While looking for tubal patency, it is important to assess that the peritoneal spillage is free and the extravasated contrast has unimpeded access to pelvic peritoneal folds and is seen to delineate the region of POD. Mere extravasation of injected contrast into the peritoneal cavity does not establish tubal normalcy. This may also happen with localized peritoneal spillage in patients with peri-tubal adhesions in the region of fimbria and should be differentiated from free spillage.

Apart from tubal patency, evaluation of tubal mucosa is an important component of tubal evaluation in HSG. Infective or inflammatory processes are likely to cause mucosal abnormality in the ampullary region with consequent formation of hydrosalpinx. The normal linear mucosal fold pattern on HSG may be replaced by cobblestone appearance. Salpingitis isthmica nodosa (SIN) is associated with infertility or pelvic inflammatory disease (PID) including tuberculosis, which is an important cause in India. SIN appears as small outpouchings or diverticula from the isthmic portion of the fallopian tube and can affect one or both tubes. Beaded appearance of fallopian tubes is often suggestive of tubercular etiology.

Apart from the tubal opacification and luminal caliber, the course of fallopian tubes should also be carefully evaluated as it provides vital clues about the status of peri-tubal peritoneum. Vertical convoluted course of fallopian tubes, clubbed lateral tubal ends, and peri-tubal halo are important determinants of peri-tubal adhesions (Fig. 7.18a–d). Contrary to popular belief, HSG does provide vital clues about the presence or absence of peri-tubal adhesions. Vertical convoluted course of fallopian tubes with peri-tubal "halo," intraperitoneal loculation, ampullary dilatation, "clubbed" distal tubal ends, fixed latero-deviation of uterus, and immobile tubes are suggested to be important determinants of peri-tubal adhesions [20, 21]. Despite its high specificity in the assessment of tubal patency, the HSG diagnosis of peri-tubal adhesions was not reported to be reliable [22]. As of today, pelvic peritoneal adhesions can be most reliably diagnosed with CT and MRI [23]. Apart from this, the course of fallopian tubes on HSG provides useful indirect clues to suspect pelvic pathologies which may be further confirmed on ultrasound or MRI.

HSG may be advised for documentation of the tubal occlusion following tubal ligation, which is seen as an abrupt termination of the tube at the surgical site or mild bulbous expansion of the tube with cutoff. New irreversible occlusion device called Essure (Conceptus, San Carlos, Calif) was introduced for minimally invasive tubal occlusion. The soft, flexible microinsert is placed hysteroscopically into each fallopian tube, which induces scar tissue formation and consequent tubal occlusion [24]. HSG may also be performed to demonstrate tubal patency without extravasation of contrast material after reversal of a ligation procedure.

Tubal polyps are rare and represent ectopic endometrial tissue located in the interstitial portion of the tube. Tubal polyps may be seen as unilateral or bilateral smooth, rounded filling defects without concomitant dilatation or tubal occlusion and are less than 1 cm in diameter. Women with tubal polyps are asymptomatic, and the association of these polyps with infertility has not been established [25].

HSG evaluation of fallopian tubes should extend beyond peritoneal spillage and tubal patency. It is important to carefully evaluate the tubal mucosal pattern, course, and caliber of the tube on each side. The peritoneal spillage should be carefully evaluated to differentiate between free and loculated spillage. Careful inspection and schematic image interpretation of HSG films may offer valuable information about the status of peritoneal cavity apart from the endometrial and tubal information in patients with infertility.

7.10.1 Therapeutic Procedures During HSG

Selective salpingography is a fluoroscopy-guided transcervical selective cannulation of the fallopian tubes, which is useful in the differentiation of cornual block and tubal spasm. The procedure offers finer tubal evaluation in terms of luminal and mucosal details and intraluminal pathology and helps to resolve discrepancy between HSG and laparoscopy. Fallopian tube recanalization (FTR) is a safe treatment option in patients with infertility from proximal tubal obstruction. The procedure involves transcervical selective cannulation of fallopian tubes to recanalize the tubal obstruction in proximal tubes. This is reported to have high technical success rate (71–92%), low complication rate, and increased chances of pregnancy (approximately 30%) and should be preferred before attempting more expensive and resource-intensive procedures. The combination of selective salpingography with fallopian tube recanalization has improved the overall management of infertility caused by tubal obstruction [26, 27].

Proximal tubal occlusion (PTO) occurs in 10–25% of women with tubal disease and is mainly due to salpingitis isthmica nodosa (SIN), chronic salpingitis, intratubal endometriosis, amorphous material (due to menstrual debris), or spasm [28]. Luminal occlusion due to menstrual debris is the primary cause in a significant number of patients with PTO. The occlusion is usually not associated with mural inflammation or peri-tubal disease. Selective salpingography and fallopian tube recanalization are therefore likely to be more effective in this group of patients with PTO. A meta-analysis has suggested that selective salpingography and transcervical cannulation under fluoroscopic guidance are effective at establishing patency in appropriately selected patients and are less invasive and costly than the surgical alternatives [29].

7.10.2 Reporting Format for Hysterosalpingography

HSG report should essentially include detailed description of the procedure including instrumentation, medications, fluoroscopy time, and radiation dosage. The status of uterus, fallopian tubes on each side, and peri-tubal adhesions should be mentioned. A standard reporting format is illustrated in Table 7.1.

Table 7.1 Standard reporting format

Procedure Medication Fluoroscopy time Radiation dose	Hysterosalpingography was performed using a metal cannula. The cervical cannulation was uneventful. The pre-procedural medication used for the procedure included oral administration of Meftal Spas 500 mg. No intra-procedural medication was administered. Pre- and post-procedural antibiotics were advised. The total fluoroscopy time is 1.01 min. The radiation dosage during the study is 192 cGy/cm cm
Endometrial cavity	Uterus is in midline location and the endometrial cavity appears normal in shape and volume with normal margins. No evidence of any definite filling defect or marginal irregularity. Mild peri-cornual venous intravasation on the left side (on later spots only) appears nonspecific
Uterine cornu	The uterine cornu appears normal on both sides
Right tube	The right fallopian tube shows normal course. There is generalized dilation of the right tube, more pronounced in the distal aspect. The ampullary mucosal folds are not visualized on right side. There is no peritoneal spillage on the right side
Left tube	The left fallopian tube shows normal course and caliber. The normal ampullary mucosal folds are visualized on the left side. There is free peritoneal spillage on the left side
Endocervical canal	The endocervical region does not reveal any definite abnormality
Pull-release	*The pull-release maneuver does not reveal any definite abnormality*
Miscellaneous	*The bones under view do not reveal any definite abnormality*

7.10.3 Sono-Hysterosalpingography (Sono-HSG)

Ultrasound-guided sono-HSG or saline infusion salpingography (SIS) in conjunction with transvaginal ultrasound is a safe, effective, and convenient diagnostic procedure for the evaluation of female genital tract. It is a suitable alternative to conventional HSG, avoiding the risks of ionizing radiation and the need to inject an iodinated contrast. It provides similar diagnostic results, perhaps with improved sensitivity and specificity for endometrial lesions [30, 31].

Sono-HSG is the preferred mode of imaging for uterine abnormalities for both primary and secondary infertility, and for evaluation of endometrium in the perimenopausal and postmenopausal age group. Common indications are irregular menstrual bleeding, recurrent miscarriage, and to check for the patency of fallopian tubes or for a baseline scan before planning IVF procedures. Endometrial polyps, intracavitary fibroids, uterine adhesions, or synechiae uterine septae are well demonstrated. Absolute contraindication of the procedure is pregnancy or suspected pregnancy. Relative contraindications are pelvic infections or unexplained pelvic tenderness.

7.10.4 Technique

- The procedure is usually performed between days 4 and 11 of the menstrual cycle.
- For perimenopausal and postmenopausal bleeding, it is performed on any day of the cycle to evaluate the cause of abnormal bleeding.

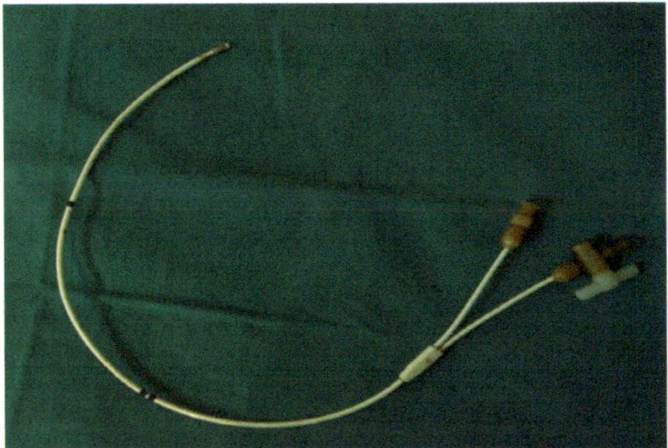

Fig. 7.15 Photograph showing a plastic cannula used for sono-HSG

Pain relief with nonsteroidal anti-inflammatory tablets (NSAID) is offered the previous night and another 2 h prior to the procedure to prevent cramping pain during catheter insertion.

Preliminary pelvic scan is performed first, both transabdominal and transvaginal to evaluate the uterus, adnexa, ovaries, and adjacent pelvic structures. The urinary bladder is emptied again just before the procedure, written informed consent is taken, and patient is placed in lithotomy position. Transvaginal probe is prepared along with the catheter guide [32]. A speculum is placed and a small thin (usually 8 or 12 French) catheter (Fig. 7.15) is inserted gently into the uterine cavity through the cervical os, through which normal saline is injected via a syringe. A sagittal view of the uterus and endometrium is focused and an initial amount of 2 mL is injected to check placement. The tip of the catheter is then inflated to retain placement. Further 20 mL or more (20–40 mL) of agitated normal saline is injected. Agitated saline produces air bubbles and improves visualization of the fallopian tubes. On real-time scan fluid is seen to distend the endometrial cavity and appears hypoechoic with a clear demarcation of the separated endometrial stripe. Endometrial lesions like polyps are then well delineated with the improved contrast between the hypoechoic fluid and hyperechoic endometrial lining. Thin endometrial adhesions are well recognized and may even be lysed by the saline. Further the probe is focused on the cornu of uterus in the transverse plane and agitated saline is pushed, to check patency, which is depicted by the stream of air and fluid bubbles exiting the cornu into the pelvic cavity. The procedure is repeated to check the patency of contralateral fallopian tube. The endometrial cavity is scanned thoroughly in both longitudinal and transverse directions. Images are annotated and saved for documentation, if required.

7.10.5 Precautions and Complications

Pregnancy test must be done to exclude pregnancy.

Before injecting the saline into the uterine cavity, the air must be cleared from the syringe by flushing a stream of saline.

Normal saline used is prewarmed or brough to room temperature, and not used cold straight from refrigerator.

Saline backflow is prevented by inflating the catheter balloon to occlude the internal cervical os. Slight pelvic discomfort during catheter insertion is usually transient and subsides in a few hours.

Routine tablet of NSAID ibuprofen is advised 1–2 h before the procedure, to relax the muscles and for pain relief.

Any post-procedural bleeding is usually related to the underlying pathophysiology and the patient is advised to bring a pad for the same. Very rarely, in less than 1% of cases there may be excessive bleeding, pain, or infection, which is treated accordingly. Antibiotics may be prescribed prophylactically, if there is a history of preceding infection.

7.10.6 Image Interpretation

Normal endometrium with sono-HSG expands symmetrically with saline instillation and appears smooth with almost similar thickness measurements on both the sides (Fig. 7.16).

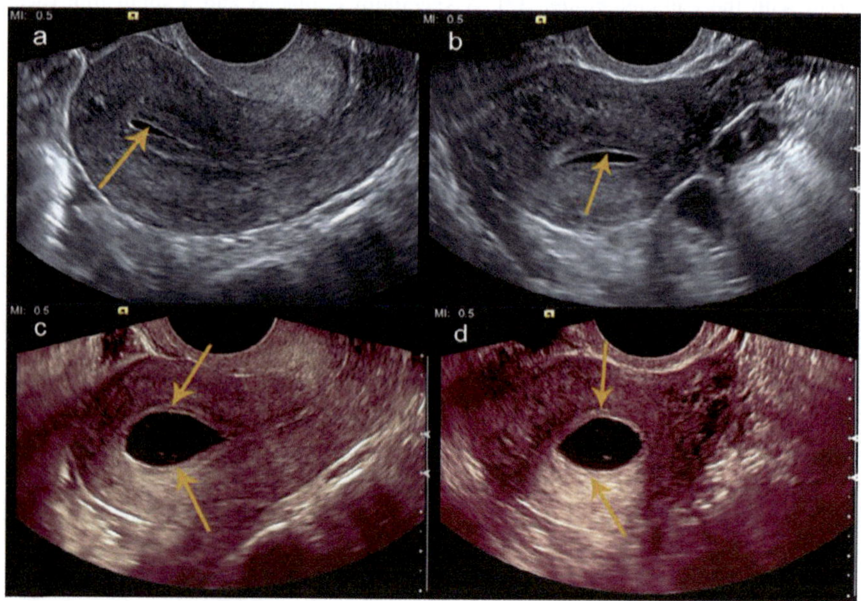

Fig. 7.16 Longitudinal (**a**, **c**) and transverse (**b**, **d**) transvaginal saline infusion sono-HSG images. Images (**a**, **b**) with minimal (5 mL) saline infusion and images (**c**, **d**) with further (20 mL) saline infusion showing well-expanded endometrial cavity (arrows) with normal smooth, symmetrical outline on both sides (acknowledgements: Dr. Shradha Chaudhary, Dept. of Gynecology, Medanta Medicity, Gurugram, Delhi NCR)

Endometrial adhesions may appear as thin or thick echogenic bands across the endometrial cavity and are well distended against the background of hypoechoic saline. The distension of the endometrial cavity may also be compromised with severe adhesions in patients with Asherman's disease (Fig. 7.17).

Endometrial polyps and submucosal fibroids are well delineated with a layer of saline, polyps generally being isoechoic to the endometrium and mucosal fibroids being hypoechoic as compared to endometrium (Figs. 7.18a, b and 7.19). Submucosal fibroids are usually broad based as compared to endometrial polyps and show distal shadowing.

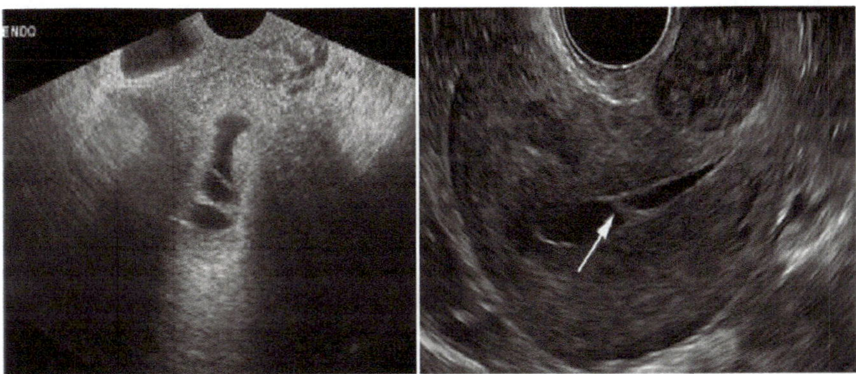

Fig. 7.17 Adhesions characteristically appear as "bridging bands" of tissue that distort the cavity. Filmy adhesions are described as thin, undulating membranes

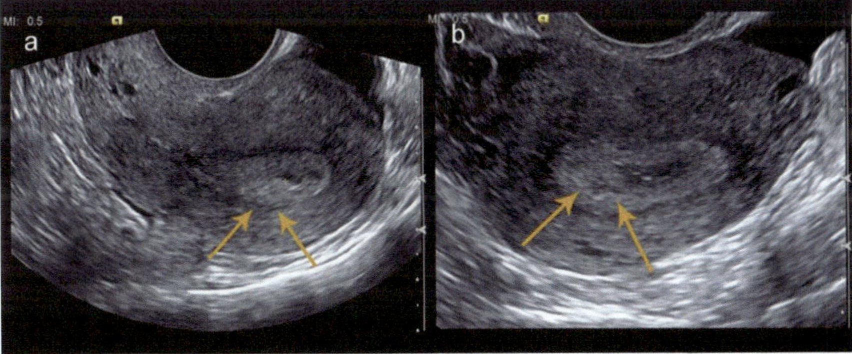

Fig. 7.18 (**a**, **b**) Longitudinal (**a**) and transverse (**b**) transvaginal sono-HSG images. Infusion of minimal (5 mL) saline infusion showing slightly demarcated hyperechoic area (arrows) in the endometrial cavity which was confirmed on hysteroscopy to be a sessile endometrial polyp. The patient clinically presented with primary infertility and intermenstrual spotting. Only minimal saline could be injected due to pain. Poor distension of the endometrial cavity also suggested endometrial adhesions in this patient (acknowledgements: Dr. Shradha Chaudhary, Dept. of Gynecology, Medanta Medicity, Gurugram, Delhi NCR)

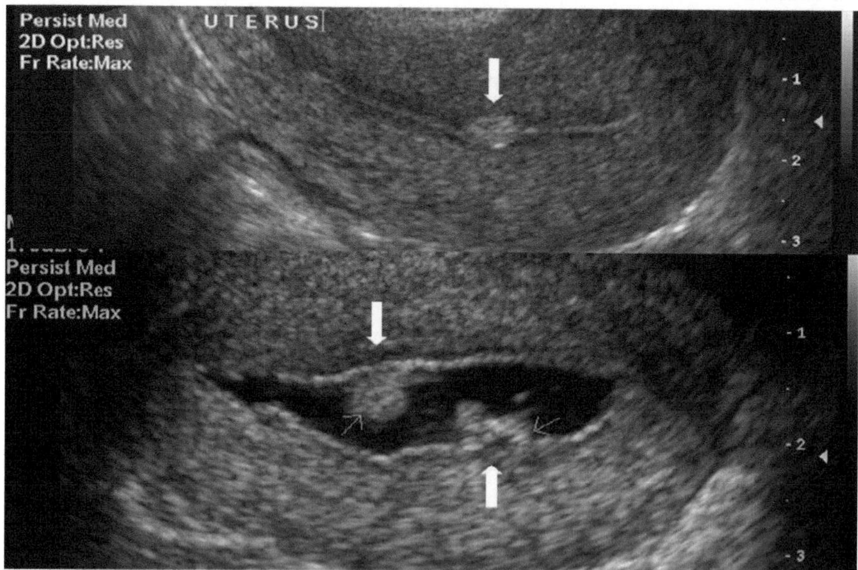

Fig. 7.19 Sono-HSG longitudinal images show focal echogenic thickening seen on transvaginal ultrasound image [arrow in upper panel]. Sono-HSG image (done in the same sitting) showing multiple focal endometrial polyps (arrows in lower panel). Optimal distension of the endometrial cavity ruled out endometrial adhesions in this patient

Diffuse endometrial pathologies such as endometrial hyperplasia may show irregularly thickened endometrial lining (Fig. 7.20a, b). Endometrial carcinoma may present as a focal or diffuse abnormality (Fig. 7.21). There is small but real risk of malignant cell dissemination in patients with endometrial carcinoma who undergo SIS. Adenomyosis may reveal loss of endometrial myometrial interface along with tiny sub-endometrial anechoic cysts [33].

7.11 Hysterosalpingo-Contrast Sonography (HyCoSy)

A further extension of SIS is HyCoSy [34] using a contrast, either SonoVue or a mixture of air and saline to test for tubal patency. With the scan focused in the transverse plane at the level of cornu, further 20 mL of agitated normal saline is injected and the spill of the contents from the cornual regions into the pelvis is then observed. There is scintillating effect noted due to the flow of echogenic air and saline from the distal end of fallopian tube into the pelvis. The spill is very transient, lasting for 5–10 s; hence the probe positioning must be appropriate to be able to observe the same and record it.

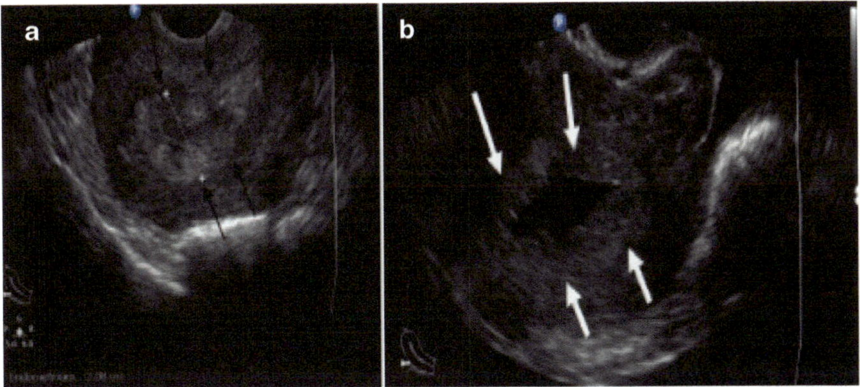

Fig. 7.20 (**a**) Shows TVS image of thickened endometrium. (**b**) Shows SIS image of endometrial hyperplasia

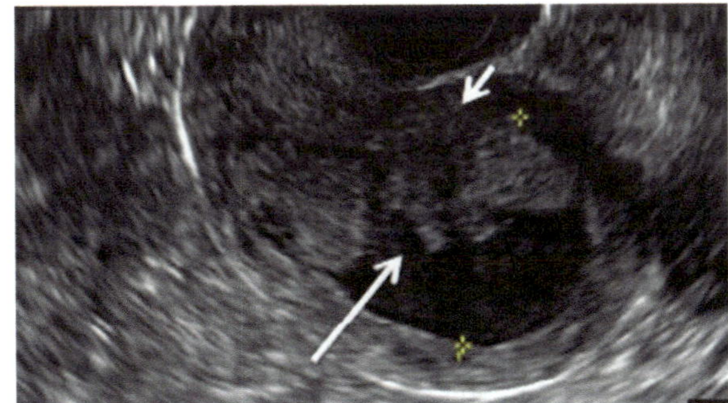

Fig. 7.21 Endometrial carcinoma may present as an irregular focal or diffuse

7.11.1 Advantages Over Conventional HSG

There are definite advantages of sono-HSG in terms of patient safety comfort and convenience to the patient.

The main advantage of sono-HSG is that it can be employed as an integrated procedure along with routine transvaginal ultrasound to evaluate the patency of fallopian tubes and other structural abnormalities, by using a single ultrasound-guided and radiation-free procedure. Use of a continuous saline air device may produce technically better image quality in sono-HSG procedures.

7.11.2 MRI and MR-HSG

Due to excellent soft-tissue resolution, MRI is accepted as the gold standard in the evaluation of the female pelvis. In terms of uterine assessment, MRI is particularly useful in the evaluation of uterine myometrium. Routine MRI offers limited information about the status of fallopian tubes and cannot evaluate tubal patency. Dynamic MR-HSG combines the advantages of HSG and MRI in a single study and allows the assessment of the uterus, patency of fallopian tubes, and extrauterine pelvic structures in a "one-stop" investigation [35]. Clinically available MR angiographic sequence (3D time-resolved imaging of contrast kinetics [TRICKS]) is reported to have high accuracy in the evaluation of tubal patency using dilute 1:100 gadodiamide and saline [36]. The technique offers adequate spatial resolution for visualization of fallopian tube contrast spillage, with superior temporal resolution of approximately 2 s per phase. This temporal resolution allows documentation of progressive spillage from left and right tubes and allows discrimination of contrast spill from the separate tubes.

7.11.3 CT-HSG

MDCT-virtual HSG is described as an additional imaging investigation that combines the advantages of HSG and MDCT imaging in female patients with infertility [37]. MDCT has high spatial resolution, which provides excellent delineation of the tubal lumen and patency when combined with HSG. MDCT-virtual HSG uses plastic cannula for instillation of the contrast medium through the cervix using the power injector. This helps to ensure a steady low pressure of instillation, and the administration of a diluted water-soluble contrast medium. MDCT-virtual HSG is therefore less painful, more comfortable, and more easily tolerated by patients than conventional HSG.

Moreover, the high spatial resolution and range of post-processing algorithms available in MDCT imaging allow precise characterization of elevated or polypoidal lesions of different sizes which is otherwise not possible without hysteroscopy. Virtual endoscopic navigation allows visualization of the inner tubal lumen. Volume rendering method provides excellent definition of the tubes and tubal pathology.

The use of 128-row MDCT allows the study to be completed in only 4 s, capturing the images in real time while the contrast is still in the tubal lumen. MDCT-virtual HSG is accurate in the diagnosis of uterine and ovarian infertility causes, while less accurate in the diagnosis of tubal causes. The sensitivity for detection of uterine and fallopian tube abnormality on MDCT-VHSG was reported to be 100% and 100%, respectively, while the specificity was reported to be 100% and 85.71%, respectively [38].

The procedure is, however, still not popular due to concerns about the effects of radiation at hysterosalpingography and pelvic MDCT [39, 40].

7.12 Clinical Recommendations

The diagnostic accuracy of HSG has been compared with that of laparoscopy and dye in a systematic review of 20 studies that distinguished between tubal obstruction and peri-tubal adhesions [22]. However, only three studies involved judgment of laparoscopy without knowledge of HSG results. Meta-analysis based on these three studies gave pooled estimates of sensitivity and specificity for HSG as a test for tubal obstruction of 0.65 (95% CI 0.50–0.78) and 0.83 (95% CI 0.77–0.88), respectively. HSG could be used as a screening test for couples with no history of pelvic infection, and if abnormal, confirmatory laparoscopy would follow [41, 42].

Considerable inter-observer variability in the interpretation of HSGs has been reported, depending on the type of pathology being assessed. Women with possible comorbidity such as pelvic and tubal diseases may need a laparoscopic assessment.

It is estimated that tubal damage accounts for 14% of fertility problems, one which suggests that when HSG suggests the presence of tubal obstruction this will be confirmed by laparoscopy in only 38% of women. Thus, HSG is a not a reliable indicator of tubal occlusion. However, when HSG suggests that the tubes are patent, this will be confirmed at laparoscopy in 94% of women, and so HSG is a reliable indicator of tubal patency [43].

Key Points

1. Hysterosalpingography (HSG) is a useful screening outpatient radiological procedure for diagnosis and has 75% sensitivity, 95% specificity, 50% positive predictive value (PPV), and 98% negative predictive value (NPV).
2. HSG is an important screening modality for evaluation of the endometrial cavity which often requires further evaluation with ultrasound, sono-HSG, or hysteroscopy.
3. HSG and sono-HSG remain important investigations in a wide range of clinical conditions including endometrial adhesions in Asherman's syndrome.
4. Intrauterine filling defects are seen in intrauterine adhesions, endometrial polyps, myomas, endometrial hyperplasia, and endometrial carcinoma.
5. Due attention to the procedural details and optimal image interpretation is certainly the key to derive the benefits of HSG and sono-HSG in these patients.

References

1. Simpson WL Jr, Beitia LG, Mester J. Hysterosalpingography: a reemerging study. Radio Graphics. 2006;26:419–31.
2. Krysiewicz S. Infertility in women: diagnostic evaluation with hysterosalpingography and other imaging techniques. AJR. 1992;159:253–61.
3. Thurmond AS. Hysterosalpingography: imaging and intervention—RSNA categorical course in genitourinary radiology. Chicago: Radiological Society of North America; 1994. p. 221–8.
4. Úbeda B, Paraira M, Alert E, Abuin RA. Hysterosalpingography: spectrum of normal variants and non-pathologic findings. AJR. 2001;177:131–5.
5. Ghonge NP, et al. Hystero-salpingography: an obituary or a new beginning …? IJRI. 2008;18(2):175–7.
6. ACR practice parameters for performance of Hysterosalpingography. Revised 2017 (Resolution 8). https://www.acr.org/-/media/ACR/Files/Practice-Parameters/HSG.pdf?la=en
7. Lindheim SR, Sprague C, Winter TC III. Hysterosalpingography and sonohysterography: lessons in technique. AJR. 2006;186:24–9.

8. Cengiz M, Kafali H, Artuc H, Baysal Z. Opioid analgesia for hysterosalpingography: controlled double-blind prospective trial with remifentanil and placebo. Gynecol Obstet Investig. 2006;62(3):168–72.
9. Liberty G, Gal M, Halevy-Shalem T, Michaelson-Cohen R, Galoyan N, Hyman J, Eldar-Geva T, Vatashsky E, Margalioth E. Lidocaine–Prilocaine (EMLA) cream as analgesia for hysterosalpingography: a prospective, randomized, controlled, double blinded study. Hum Reprod. 2007;22(5):1335–9.
10. Karasick S. Hysterosalpingography. Urol Radiol. 1991;13:67–73.
11. Rasmussen F, Lindequist S, Larsen C, Justessen F. Therapeutic effect of hysterosalpingography: oil- versus water-soluble contrast media—a randomized prospective study. Radiology. 1991;179:75–8.
12. Alper MM, Garner PR, Spence JEH, Quarrington AM. Pregnancy rates after hysterosalpingography with oil- and water-soluble contrast media. Obstet Gynecol. 1986;68:6–9.
13. Dreyer K, Rijswijk JV, Mijatovic V, Goddijn M, Verhoeve H, Rooij IA, et al. Oil-based or water-based contrast for hysterosalpingography in infertile women. N Engl J Med. 2017;376:2043–52.
14. Perisinakis K, Damilakis J, Grammatikakis J, Theocharopoulos N, Gourtsoyiannis N. Radiogenic risks from hysterosalpingography. EurRadiol. 2003 Jul;13(7):1522–8.
15. General Radiation Safety; Standard guidelines. www.imagewisely.org.
16. Atomic Energy (Radiation Protection) Rules 2004. AERB guidelines. https://aerb.gov.in/images/PDF/DiagnosticRadiology/e-LORA-Diagnostic-Radiology-Guidelines.pdf.
17. The American Fertility Society. Classifications of adnexal adhesions, distal tubal occlusion, tubal occlusion secondary to tubal ligation, tubal pregnancies, müllerian anomalies and intrauterine adhesions. Fertil Steril. 1988;49(6):944–55.
18. Behr SC, Courtier JL, Qayyum A. Imaging of Müllerian duct anomalies. Radiographics. 2012;32:E233–50.
19. Winfield AC, Pittaway D, Maxson W, Daniell J, Wentz AC. Apparent cornual occlusion in hysterosalpingography: reversal by glucagon. AJR Am J Roentgenol. 1982;139:525–7.
20. Karasick S, Goldfarb AF. Peritubal adhesions in infertile women: diagnosis with hysterosalpingography. AJR Am J Roentgenol. 1989;152(4):777–9.
21. Wu D-D, Niu Z-H, Zhang A-J, Guy R-H, Feng UN. An impact of suspected peritubal adhesions by hysterosalpingography on outcomes of intrauterine insemination. J Reprod Contracept. 2013;24(3):173–80.
22. Swart P, Mol BWJ, van der Veen F, van Beurden M, Redekop WK, Bossuyt PMM. The accuracy of hysterosalpingography in the diagnosis of tubal pathology: a meta-analysis. Fertil Steril. 1995;64:3.
23. Ghonge NP, Ghonge Sanchita D. Computed tomography and magnetic resonance imaging in the evaluation of pelvic peritoneal adhesions: What radiologists need to know? Ind J Radiol Imag. 2014;24:149–55.
24. Essure home page. www.Essure.com. Accessed 18 Oct 2004.
25. Ubeda B, Paraira M, Alert E, Abuin RA. Hysterosalpingography: spectrum of normal variants and nonpathological findings. AJR Am J Roentgenol. 2001;177(1):131–5.
26. Thurmond AS, Machan LS, Maubon AJ, Rouanet J-P, Hovsepian DM, Van Moore A, Zagoria RJ, Dickey KW, Bass JC. A review of selective salpingography and fallopian tube catheterization. Radiographics. 2000;20:1759–68.
27. Anil G, Tay KH, Loh SF, Yong TT, Ong CL, Tan BS. Fluoroscopy-guided, transcervical, selective salpingography and fallopian tube recanalisation. J Obstet Gynaecol. 2011;31(8):746–50.
28. Sulak PJ, Letterie GS, Coddington CC, Hayslip CC, Woodward JE, Klein TA. Histology of proximal tubal occlusion. Fertil Steril. 1987;48:437–40.
29. Honore´ GM, AEC H, Schenken RS. Pathophysiology and management of proximal tubal blockage. Fertil Steril. 1999;71:5.
30. Maheux-Lacroix S, Boutin A, Moore L, Bergeron M-E, Bujold E, Laberge P, Lemyre M, Dodin S. Hysterosalpingosonography for diagnosing tubal occlusion in sub fertile women: a systematic review with meta-analysis. Hum Reprod. 2014;29(5):953–63.

31. Acholonu UC, Silberzweig J, Stein DE, Keltz M. Hysterosalpingography versus sonohysterography for intrauterine abnormalities. JSLS. 2011;15(4):471–4.
32. AIUM Practice Guideline for the Performance of Sonohysterography. Guideline developed in collaboration with the American College of Radiology, American College of Obstetricians and Gynecologists, Society of Radiologists in Ultrasound. J Ultrasound Med. 2015;34:1.
33. Yang T, Pandya A, Marcal L, Bude RO, Platt JF, Bedi DG, Elsayes KM. Sonohysterography: principles, technique and role in diagnosis of endometrial pathology. World J Radiol. 2013;5(3):81–7.
34. Saunders RD, Shwayder JM, Nakajima ST. Current methods of tubal patency assessment. Fertil Steril. 2011;95:2171–9.
35. Winter L, Glücker T, Steimann S, Fröhlich JM, Steinbrich W, Geyter CD, Pegios W. Feasibility of dynamic MR hysterosalpingography for the diagnostic work-up of infertile women. Acta Radiol. 2010;51(6):693–701.
36. Sadowski EA, Ochsner JE, Riherd JM, Korosec FR, Agrawal G, Pritts EA, Kliewer MA. MR hysterosalpingography with an angiographic time-resolved 3D pulse sequence: assessment of tubal patency. AJR. 2008;191:1381–5.
37. Carrascosa PM, Capuñay C, Vallejos J, Martín López EB, Baronio M, Carrascosa JM. Virtual hysterosalpingography: a new multidetector CT technique for evaluating the female reproductive system. Radiographics. 2010;30:643–63.
38. Hasan DI, Mohammad FF, Shazely S. Utility of 128-multislice CT virtual HSG in assessment of female infertility. Egypt J Radiol Nucl Med. 2016;47:1743–52.
39. Fernández JM, Vañó E, Guibelalde E. Patient doses in hysterosalpingography. Br J Radiol. 1996;69(824):751–4.
40. Huda W, Vance A. Patient radiation doses from adult and pediatric CT. AJR Am J Roentgenol. 2007;188(2):540–6.
41. Collins JA. Diagnostic assessment of the infertile female partner. Curr Probl Obstet Gynecol Fertil. 1988;11:6–42.
42. Opsahl MS, Miller B, Klein TA. The predictive value of hysterosalpingography for tubal and peritoneal infertility factors. Fertil Steril. 1993;60:444–8.
43. Fertility: assessment and treatment for people with fertility problems. NICE Clinical Guideline February 2013. 2nd edition; 2013 National Collaborating Centre for Women's and Children's Health.

Diagnostic Hysteroscopy

8

Sergio Haimovich

The diagnosis of intrauterine adhesion and hence Asherman syndrome (AS) can sometimes be missed.

Several diagnostic modalities have been evaluated for the diagnosis of intrauterine adhesions (IUAs). IUA can be visualized by hysterosalpingography (HSG), ultrasonography including contrast sonohysterography (SHG), 3D ultrasonography, hysteroscopy, and magnetic resonance imaging (MRI).

Hysteroscopy is the gold standard in studies comparing different diagnostic modalities, and several classification systems are based on hysteroscopic findings.

The technique of ***"vaginoscopy" introduced by Stefano Bettocchi in 1997*** has revolutionized office hysteroscopy.

Vaginoscopy has been described in the literature as far back as the 1950s and continues to be used for diagnosing vaginal endometriosis, pelvic floor mesh erosions, vaginal fistulas, and cervical pathology, for example, as well as excising vaginal lesions or longitudinal vaginal septum. It has also been utilized in the pediatric/adolescent population for visualizing and removing for eigenbodies, and for evaluating pelvic trauma, abnormal bleeding, and infection.

Dr. Stefano Bettocchi and Dr. Luigi Selvaggi in Italy were the first, however, to describe the utilization of a vaginoscopic approach to office hysteroscopy for evaluating the endocervical canal and uterine cavity in addition to the vagina and external cervical os. In a paper published in 1997 in the Journal of the American Association of Gynecologic Laparoscopists (4:255–8), they described various approaches they took to improve patient tolerance during the 1200 diagnostic hysteroscopies they performed between 1992 and 1996.

S. Haimovich (✉)
Head of the Hysteroscopy Unit, Del Mar University Hospital, Barcelona, Spain

Director of the Gynecology Ambulatory Surgery Unit, Hillel Yaffe Medical Center/Rappaport Faculty of Medicine - Technion, Hadera, Israel
e-mail: sergio@haimovich.net

R. Manchanda (ed.), *Intra Uterine Adhesions*,
https://doi.org/10.1007/978-981-33-4145-6_8

8.1 Vaginoscopic Office Hysteroscopy Includes Following Points, Fig. 8.1

- No-touch technique.
- For atramautic insertion of hysteroscope into OS.
- **NO** speculum/tenaculum.
- Place hysteroscope in lower vagina, and distend it with a pressure of 30–40 mmHg.
- Move the hysteroscope in posterior fornix and visualize portio.
- Move backward to identify external os.
- Cross ext. os, and consider fore-oblique view of 12°–30° hysteroscope.
- To reduce the possible trauma during this phase, keep the scope located in the middle of the canal, avoiding stimulation of the muscle fibers.

8.1.1 Advantages of Vaginoscopy

- Vaginoscopic approach consumes equal time as conventional approach.
- Detailed evaluation of the vaginal walls, fornices, and ectocervix.
- Reduces patient discomfort.
- Allows the examination even in virgin patients, severe vaginal atrophy or stenosis.

8.2 Recommendations for Analgesics: Diagnostic Office Hysteroscopy

RCOG 2011—Tab. ibuprofen 400 mg or tab. paracetamol 1 g or any analgesic at least 1 h before the procedure

ACOG 2018

- Tab. misoprostol (off label) 200–400 μg oral or intravaginal, the night before surgery
- Pre-op NSAIDS
- Antianxiety medications

8.3 Recommendations for Analgesics: Operative Office Hysteroscopy

- Paracervical injections of local anesthetic significantly reduced pain in women undergoing outpatient hysteroscopy. Maximum dose of lidocaine is 4.5 mg/kg. 200 mg of lidocaine (20 mL of 1% lidocaine) is injected at cervicovaginal junction—2.4.6.8.10 o'clock positions at 1.5–2 mm depth.
- Combined cervical block protocols for the resection of polyps and myomas. Randomized trial found a statistically significant difference in pain score between

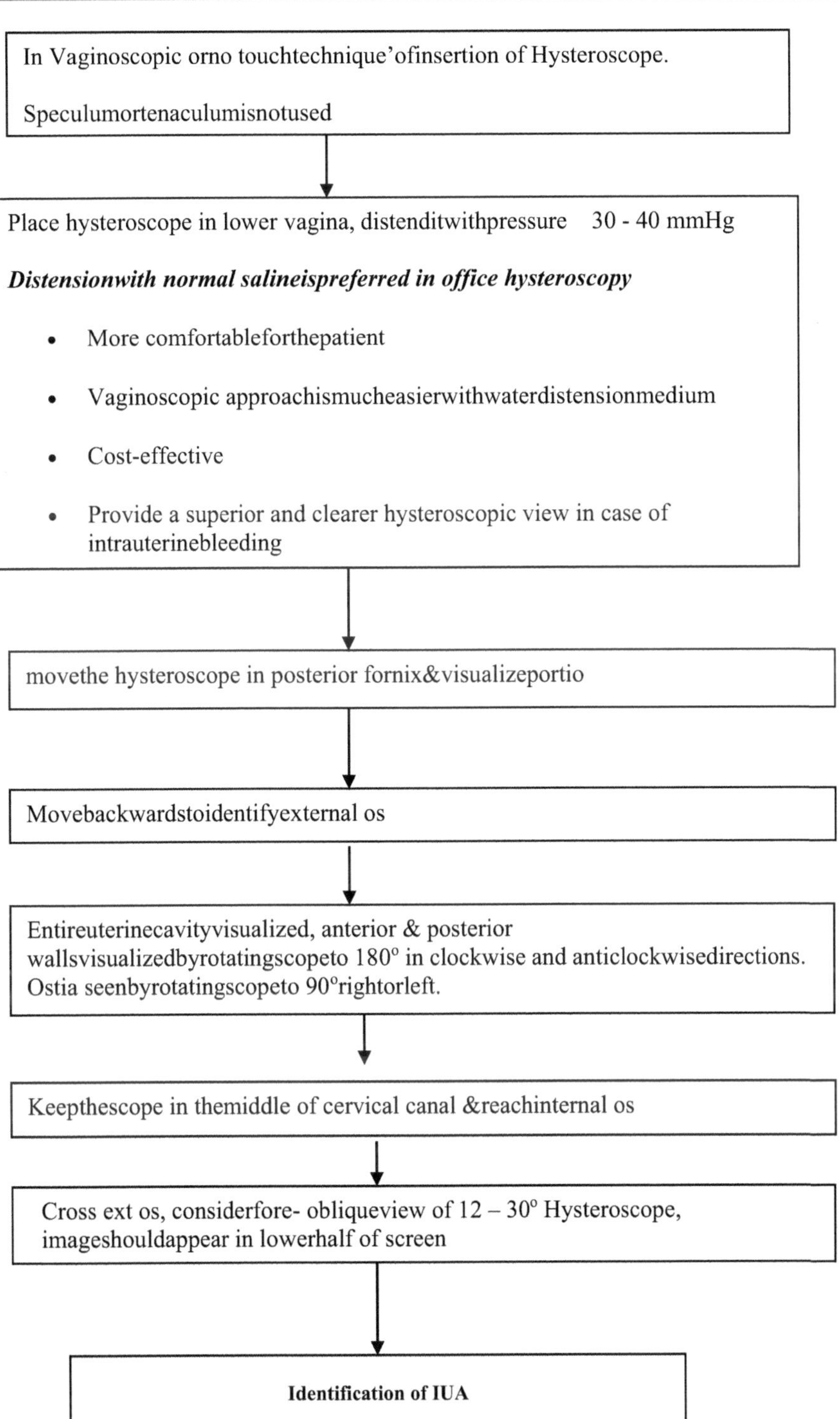

Fig. 8.1 Vaginoscopy procedure

a group receiving **paracervical and intracervical** block and the group only receiving intracervical block (*1.3 vs. 2.1, respectively*).

- Conscious sedation (0.25 mg i.v. fentanyl + 0.5 mg atropine + 2 mg midazolam) does not cause significant differences in terms of intraoperative or postoperative pain or the woman's satisfaction. Close monitoring is needed, as it can depress the CNS and has the potential to impair respiration, circulation, or both. Thus, it is not recommended.

8.3.1 Anticipated Cervical Stenosis

8.3.1.1 Medical Methods

- Misoprostol 400 mg either orally or vaginally 6–8 h prior to surgery or 400 mg sublingually 2–4 h prior to surgery.
- Hygroscopic dilators—Laminaria tents or Dilapan S (3 × 55 mm or 4 × 55 mm) 12 h before procedure.
- Intracervical injection of vasopressin solution (4 IU in 100 cm^3 sodium chloride) injected at the 4 and 8 o'clock positions.

NAM Cooper [1] (2010) conducted a systematic review of vaginoscopic procedures and its effect on pain; there were six trials (2851 participants). Data from four of these were meta-analyzed, and we found that the use of the vaginoscopic approach to hysteroscopy was less painful than using the traditional technique (SMD) 0.44, 95% CI from 0.65 to 0.22, I 2 = 58%. There was no significant difference in the number of failed procedures between groups ($P = 0.38$).

They concluded that the vaginoscopic approach to outpatient hysteroscopy is successful and significantly reduces the pain experienced by patients during the procedure, compared with traditional techniques using a vaginal speculum. Vaginoscopy should become standard practice for endoscopic instrumentation of the uterine cavity in the outpatient setting.

P.P. Smith et al. [2] (2019) reported that vaginoscopy was significantly more successful than standard hysteroscopy [647/726 (89%) versus 621/734 (85%), respectively; relative risk (RR) 1.05, 95% CI 1.01–1.10; $P = 0.01$]. The median time taken to complete vaginoscopy was 2 min compared with 3 min for standard hysteroscopy ($P < 0.001$). The mean pain score was 42.7 for vaginoscopy, which was significantly less than standard hysteroscopy 46.4 ($P = 0.02$). Operative complications occurred in 5 women receiving vaginoscopy and 19 women receiving standard hysteroscopy (RR 0.26, 95% CI 0.10–0.69).

New developments in hysteroscopes and sheath were generally dominated by decreasing outer diameter without losing the quality of the image. This is extremely important since the operating field in the (obstructed) uterine cavity in patients with AS is often very limited in space.

Any hysteroscopes or resectoscopes with outer sheath diameter up to 5 mm are called miniaturized instruments. They are less invasive, less painful, and without the need of cervical dilatation (Fig. 8.2).

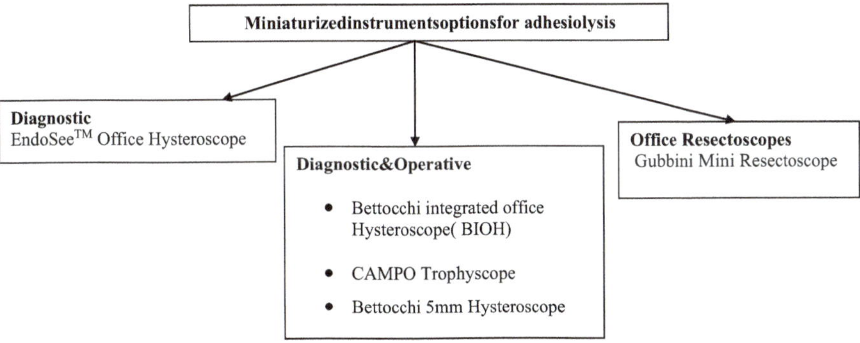

Fig. 8.2 Miniaturized instrument options for adhesiolysis

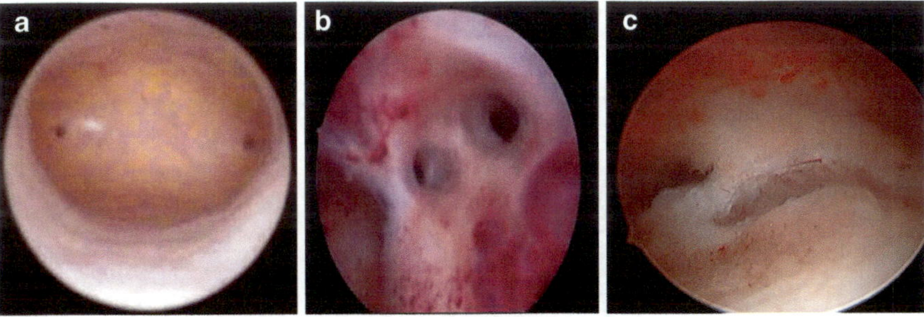

Fig. 8.3 (**a**) Normal cavity. (**b**) Mucosal adhesions are frequently pink, like the surrounding endometrium, and easy to lyse. (**c**) Fibromuscular adhesions appear as thicker, white band

During hysteroscopy, intrauterine adhesions can be visualized, and the severity of the condition assessed (Figs. 8.3, 8.4, 8.5, 8.6, 8.7, 8.8, and 8.9).

It is also possible to estimate the proportion of healthy endometrial tissue, which may help to estimate the prognosis.

Patients with cervical stenosis might benefit from the use of intravaginal misoprostol insertion the evening before hysteroscopy, ensuring that the cervical canal is easier to dilate [3, 4].

A blind dilatation should never be performed as it can destroy details like dark areas that absorb more light indicating an entrance to a (part of a) cavity or differences in color or level of depth in the obstruction that might lead to the right way to find the remaining parts of the cavity.

Contrast sonohysterography has a high negative predictive value (98%), but a moderate positive predictive value (43%) when compared with hysteroscopy [5, 6].

In a Taiwanese study of 110 women, 3D sonography was compared with hysteroscopy, finding a confirmation range of 16–100% in accordance to the number of

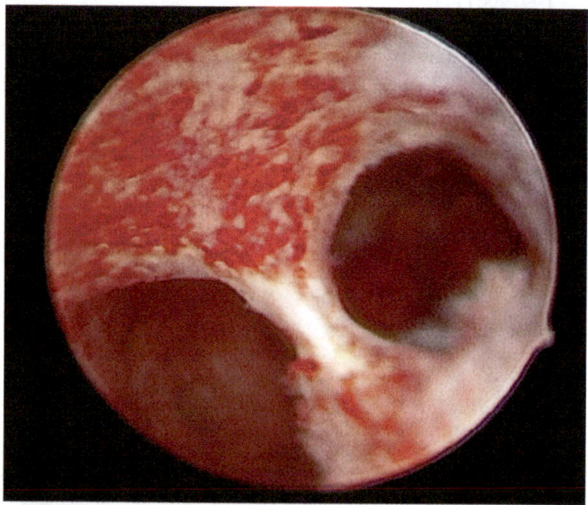

Fig. 8.4 Isthmic adhesion

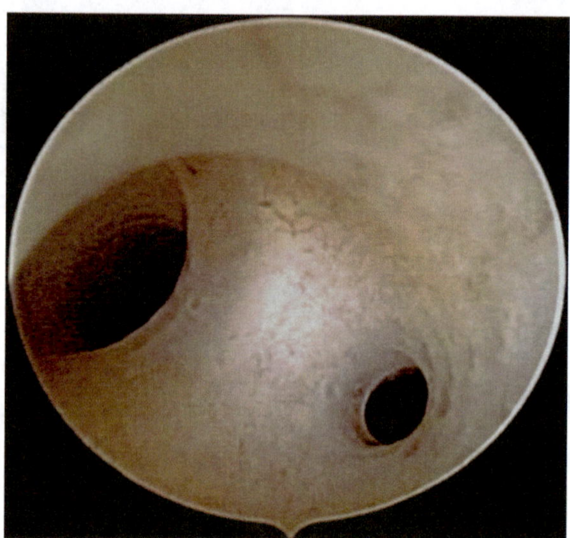

Fig. 8.5 Thick adhesion

morphological abnormalities, including marginal irregularity, thinning defects, obliteration, fibrosis, and calcification [7].

HSG, SHG, and hysteroscopy are all of limited diagnostic value when the cavity is totally obstructed. In these rare cases MRI can be valuable, although too expensive as a routine diagnostic tool.

Compared with radiologic investigations, and provided that the endometrial cavity is accessible, hysteroscopy more accurately confirms the presence, extent, and morphological characteristics of adhesions and the quality of the endometrium. It provides a real-time view of the cavity, enabling accurate description of location and degree of adhesions, classification, and concurrent treatment of IUAs [8].

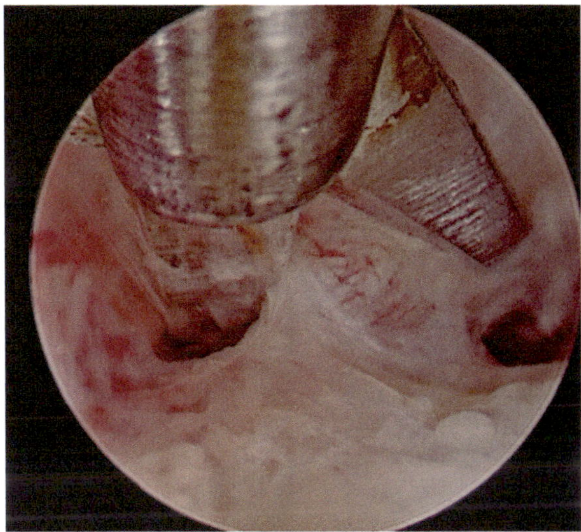

Fig. 8.6 Cutting an isthmic adhesion

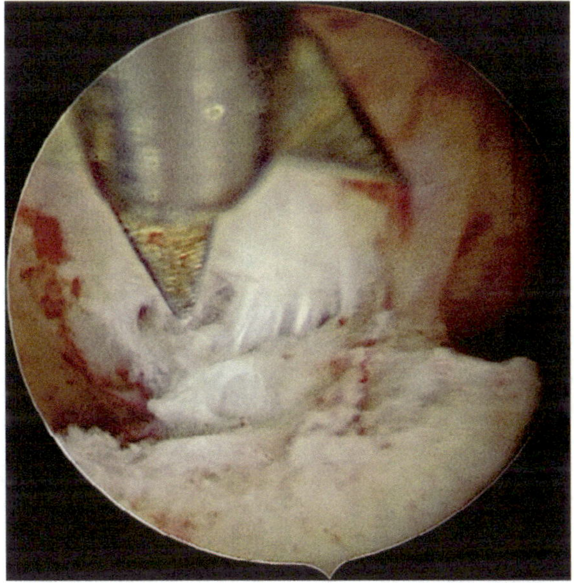

Fig. 8.7 Notice the fibrotic tissue of the adhesion

In difficult cases the simultaneous guidance of an ultrasound will be necessary [9, 10].

It can be used to demonstrate an area of proliferated endometrium in the upper part of the uterine cavity.

Some authors favor laparoscopy to decrease the risk of perforation; however, laparoscopy will not prevent perforation.

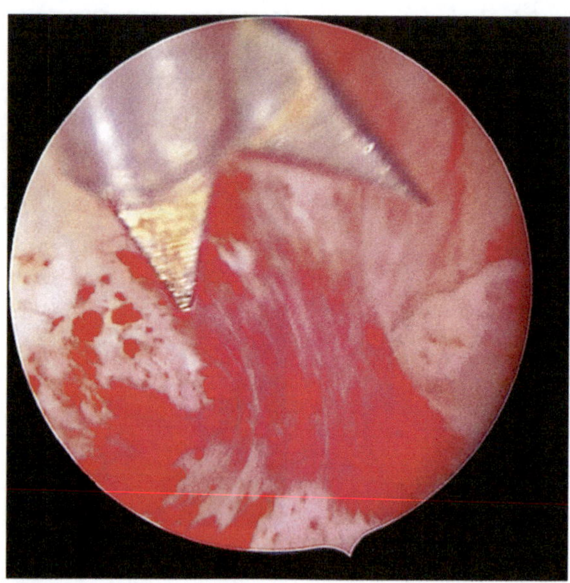

Fig. 8.8 Fundal adhesion

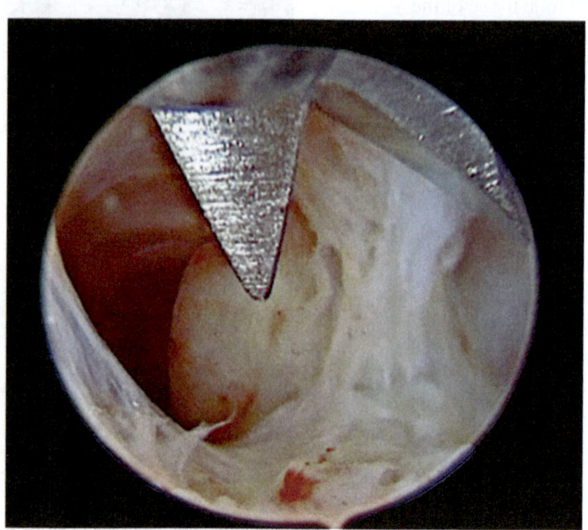

Fig. 8.9 Anteroposterior adhesion

Perforation of the uterus is a well-known complication of difficult hysteroscopic surgery.

In almost all studies, hysteroscopic adhesiolysis as the treatment of AS is mentioned as the procedure with the highest incidence of perforation.

When a perforation occurs during the introduction of the hysteroscope or by a nonactivated surgical conventional instrument like forceps and scissors used in a (non-blind) visual way, intra-abdominal bleeding and intestinal perforation are very rare, and an expectative management seems justified.

Intrauterine adhesions should be classified as this can serve as a guide to the prognosis following treatment, which in itself is related to the severity of the disease [11].

Several classification systems have been proposed for the description of the severity of IUA and AS; each of them includes hysteroscopy to determine the characteristics of the adhesions. Note: Classification has been described in detail in Chap. 4.

They are all descriptive in different ways and are therefore noncomparable. Only two classification systems include symptoms regarding AS (obstetric or menstrual history). Three of the classifications [12–14] are descriptive with three stages: minimal/mild, moderate, and severe based on the hysteroscopic assessment of the extent and type of adhesions (filmy, firm/dense). Hamou et al. [15] describe the adhesions as isthmic, marginal, central, and severe.

The former European Society of Hysteroscopy [16] operated with four grades with subtypes (seven stages in all), while Donnez [17] uses six grades based on hysteroscopy and HSG with postoperative pregnancy rate as the primary driver. Finally, Nasr et al. [18] have developed a complex system with hysteroscopic assessment combined with menstrual and obstetric history. None of the used classification systems have been validated or examined in relation to reproductive performance and unfortunately no comparative analysis has been performed for the classification systems as comparisons between studies are difficult to interpret. In Table 8.1 all the classifications and the key features are summarized.

Two of the most used classification systems are:

Table 8.1 Classification of intrauterine adhesions [6]

Source	Summary of classification
March et al. [12]	Adhesions classified as minimal, moderate, or severe based on hysteroscopic assessment of the degree of uterine cavity involvement
Hamou et al. [15]	Adhesions classified as isthmic, marginal, central, or severe according to hysteroscopic assessment
Valle and Sciarra [13]	Adhesions classified as mild, moderate, or severe according to hysteroscopic assessment and extent of occlusion (partial or total) at HSG
European Society of Hysteroscopy [16]	Complex system classifies IUAs as grades I through IV with several subtypes and incorporates a combination of hysteroscopic and HSG findings and clinical symptoms
American Fertility Society [14]	Complex scored system of mild, moderate, or severe IUAs based on the extent of endometrial cavity obliteration, appearance of adhesions, and patient menstrual characteristics based on hysteroscopic or HSG assessment
Donnez and Nisolle [17]	Adhesions classified into six grades on the basis of location, with postoperative pregnancy rate as the primary driver. Hysteroscopy or HSG is used for assessment
Nasr et al. [18]	Complex system creates a prognostic score by incorporating menstrual and obstetric history with IUA findings at hysteroscopic assessment

Table 8.2 The European Society of Hysteroscopy classification of intrauterine adhesions

Grade	Extent of intrauterine adhesions
I	Thin or filmy adhesions easily ruptured by hysteroscope sheath alone, cornual areas normal
II	Singular filmy adhesions connecting separate parts of the uterine cavity, visualization of both tubal ostia possible, cannot be ruptured by hysteroscope sheath alone
IIA	Occluding adhesions only in the region of the internal cervical os. Upper uterine cavity normal
III	Multiple firm adhesions connecting separate parts of the uterine cavity, unilateral obliteration of ostial areas of the tubes
IIIA	Extensive scarring of the uterine cavity wall with amenorrhea or hypomenorrhea
IIIB	Combination of III and IIIA
IV	Extensive firm adhesions with agglutination of the uterine walls. Both tubal ostial areas occluded

The European Society of Hysteroscopy classification [16] of intrauterine adhesions which is shown in Table 8.2 and the American Society for Reproductive Medicine classification [14] of intrauterine adhesions shown in Table 8.3.

Based on the "see-and-treat" approach, although being a diagnostic tool, hysteroscopy becomes also a surgical tool.

In order to avert further damage of the endometrial lining, only conventional instruments should be used. High-frequency electrical surgical instruments (electrodes or resectoscopes) should not be used in the treatment of patients with AS. The local and lateral spread of heat and electricity could eventually destroy parts of original vital endometrial lining.

Following placement of the scope into the entrance of the endometrial cavity, hysteroscopic scissors of forceps are advanced through the operative channel and used to divide any noted adhesions. Filmy adhesions can be ruptured often by touching them with the sheath of the hysteroscope or even only by the pressure of the inflow of distension and irrigation fluid. Adhesiolysis should begin with the most centrally located adhesions and proceed to those located at the periphery of the cavity. Especially myometrial vasculature, showing the margins of the original cavity, is best recognized by the lowest intrauterine pressure and distension that allows visualization. With the use of conventional instruments like scissors and forceps, further damage to the remaining endometrial lining is prevented.

Summarized evidence based on AAGL practice report: practice guidelines on intrauterine adhesions developed in collaboration with the European Society for Gynaecological Endoscopy (ESGE) [8]:

1. Hysteroscopy is the most accurate method for diagnosis of IUAs and should be the investigation of choice when available: Level B.
2. Intrauterine adhesions should be classified as prognosis is correlated with severity of adhesions: Level B.
3. The various classification systems make comparison between studies difficult to interpret. This may reflect inherent deficiencies in each of the classification systems. Consequently, it is currently not possible to endorse any specific system: Level C.

Table 8.3 The American Society for Reproductive Medicine classification of intrauterine adhesions

Patient's name _____		Date _____		Chart_____		Chart_____	
Age _____	G _____	P _____	Sp Ab _____	VTP _____	Ectopic _____	Infertile yes _____	No _____
Other significant history (i.e., surgery, infection, etc.) ______________________________							
HSG _____		Sonography _____		Photography _____		Laparoscopy _____	Laparotomy _____
Extent of cavity involved	<1/3	1/3–2/3	>2/3				
	1	2	4				
Type of adhesions	Filmy	Filmy and dense	Dense				
	1	2	4				
Menstrual pattern	Normal	Hypomenorrhea	Amenorrhea				
	0	2	4				
Prognostic classification		HSG score	Hysteroscopy score	Additional findings			
Stage I (mild)	1–4	___	___	_______________			
Stage II (moderate)	5–8	___	___	_______________			
Stage III (severe)	9–12	___	___	_______________			

Key Points

1. Hysteroscopy is the gold standard for the diagnosis and treatment of AS.
2. The technique of "vaginoscopy" introduced by Stefano Bettocchi in 1997 has revolutionized office hysteroscopy.
3. Vaginoscopy includes no-touch technique or no speculum and tenaculum.
4. Paracervical injections of local anesthetic significantly reduced pain in women undergoing outpatient hysteroscopy.
5. Hysteroscopes or resectoscopes with outer sheath diameter up to 5 mm are called miniaturized instruments.
6. During hysteroscopy, intrauterine adhesions can be visualized, and the severity of the condition assessed. Adhesiolysis can be performed in the same sitting.

References

1. Cooper NAM, Smith P, Khan KS, Clark TJ. Vaginoscopic approach to outpatient hysteroscopy: a systematic review of the effect on pain. BJOG. 2010;117:532–9. https://doi.org/10.1111/j.1471-0528.2010.02503.X.
2. Smith PP, Kolhe S, O'Connor S, Clark TJ. Vaginoscopy against standard treatment: a randomised controlled trial. BJOG. 2019;126(7):891–9. https://doi.org/10.1111/1471-0528.15665.
3. Al-Fozan H, Firwana B, Alkadri H, Hassan S, Tulandi T. Preoperative ripening of the cervix before operative hysteroscopy. Cochrane Database Syst Rev. 2015;23(4):CD005998.
4. Oppegaard KS, Wesheim BI, Istre O, Qvigstad E. Comparison of self-administered misoprostol versus placebo for cervical ripening prior to operative hysteroscopy using a sequential design. BJOG. 2008;115(5):663e9.
5. Soares SR, Barbosa dos Reis MM, Camargos AF. Diagnostic accuracy of sonohysterography, transvaginal sonography, and hysterosalpingography in patients with uterine cavity diseases. Fertil Steril. 2000;73(2):406–11.
6. Salle B, Gaucherand P, de Saint Hilaire P, Rudigoz RC. Transvaginal sonohysterographic evaluation of intrauterine adhesions. J Clin Ultrasound. 1999;27(3):131–4.
7. Kim MJ, Lee Y, Lee C, et al. Accuracy of three dimensional ultrasound and treatment outcomes of intrauterine adhesion in infertile women. Taiwan J Obstet Gynecol. 2015;54(6):737–41.
8. AAGL Elevating Gynecologic Surgery. AAGL practice report: practice guidelines on intrauterine adhesions developed in collaboration with the European Society of Gynaecological Endoscopy (ESGE). Gynecol Surg. 2017;14:6. https://doi.org/10.1186/s10397-017-1007-3.
9. Bellingham R. Intrauterine adhesions: hysteroscopic lysis and adjunctive methods. Aust NZ J Obstet Gynaecol. 1996;36:171–4.
10. Deans R, Abbott J. Review of intrauterine adhesions. J Minim Invasive Gynecol. 2010;17:555–69.
11. Magos A. Hysteroscopic treatment of Asherman's syndrome. Reprod BioMed Online. 2002;4(Supp 3):46–51.
12. March CM, Israel R, March AD. Hysteroscopic management of intrauterine adhesions. Am J Obstet Gynecol. 1978;130(6):653–7.
13. Valle RF, Sciarra JJ. Intrauterine adhesions: hysteroscopic diagnosis, classification, treatment, and reproductive outcome. Am J Obstet Gynecol. 1988;158(6 Pt 1):1459–70.
14. The American Fertility Society. Classifications of adnexal adhesions, distal tubal occlusion, tubal occlusion secondary to tubal ligation, tubal pregnancies, Müllerian anomalies and intrauterine adhesions. Fertil Steril. 1988;49(6):944–55.
15. Hamou J, Salat-Baroux J, Siegler AM. Diagnosis and treatment of intrauterine adhesions by microhysteroscopy. Fertil Steril. 1983;39(3):321–6.

16. Wamsteker K. Diagnostic hysteroscopy: technique and documentation. In: Sutton CD, Diamond M, editors. Endoscopic surgery for gynecologists. London, UK: WB Saunders; 1998. p. 511–24.
17. Donnez J, Nisolle M. Hysteroscopic adhesiolysis of intrauterine adhesions (Asherman syndrome). In: Donnez J, editor. Atlas of laser operative laparoscopy and hysteroscopy. London, UK: Parthenon Publishing Group; 1994. p. 305–22.
18. Nasr AL, Al-Inany HG, Thabet SM, Aboulghar M. A clinic hysteroscopic scoring system of intrauterine adhesions. Gynecol Obstet Investig. 2000;50(3):178–81.

9 Overview and Treatment: Hysteroscopic Techniques

Ferdinando Murgia, Fabiana Divina Fascilla, and Stefano Bettocchi

9.1 Overview

Intrauterine adhesions have been recognized as a cause of secondary amenorrhea since the end of the nineteenth century [1].

More than a century ago, H. Fritsch [1] first reported a case of post-traumatic intrauterine adhesion and in the mid-twentieth century, Stamer [2] reviewed the literature and added 24 cases of his own with intrauterine adhesions associated with gravid uterus.

In 1948, Joseph G. Asherman further described the eponymous condition with a series of papers [3–6] about frequency, etiology, symptoms, and roentgenologic picture of this condition.

The terms “Asherman’s syndrome” (AS) and intrauterine adhesions (IUAs) are often used interchangeably, although the syndrome requires the constellation of signs and symptoms (pain, menstrual disturbance, and subfertility in any combination) related to the presence of IUAs; the presence of IUAs in the absence of symptoms is of questionable clinical significance.

Asherman’s syndrome has an impact on both reproductive outcomes and gynecologic symptoms and invariably may affect patients’ physical and psychosocial health; while understanding and preventing the causes of intrauterine adhesions are

F. Murgia
II Unit of Obstetrics and Gynecology, Department D.I.M.O., University “Aldo Moro”, Bari, Italy

F. D. Fascilla
Unit of Obstetrics and Gynecology, “Di Venere” Hospital, ASL Ba, Bari, Italy

S. Bettocchi (✉)
Inter-Departmental Project Unit of “Minimal-Invasive Gynecological Surgery”, University “Aldo Moro”, Bari, Italy
e-mail: stefano.bettocchi@uniba.it

R. Manchanda (ed.), *Intra Uterine Adhesions*,
https://doi.org/10.1007/978-981-33-4145-6_9

sometimes challenging, the correct surgical management is often successful in restoring physiology and offers favorable fertility outcomes; in retrospective cohort studies including patients with AS treated with adhesiolysis, rates of successful restoration of menses and cavity anatomy are greater than 95%.

Substantial progress has been made since the Asherman's report: large-scale series, although retrospective, have reported clinical outcomes while randomized controlled trials (RCTs) have investigated both primary and secondary adhesion prevention including solid and semisolid barriers.

Prevention of re-formation of adhesions is still debated as no single method for preventing recurrence has shown superiority while recent human studies documenting successful pregnancy outcomes after stem cell treatments following intermittent hysteroscopy are reported.

Although some new therapeutic approaches hold promise for future, hysteroscopic management with lysis of adhesions remains the gold standard for diagnosis and treatment and surely adopting an office-based approach offers several advantages.

9.2 Epidemiology

Accurate incidence of IUAs is difficult to ascertain, as few studies assess the occurrence of adhesion formation in a prospective fashion.

Another conundrum is that Asherman's syndrome may go unrecognized in women who are not trying to conceive since they may not recognize or be concerned with the symptoms such as hypomenorrhea. On the other hand, this clinical condition may be underdiagnosed because it is usually undetectable by routine examinations or diagnostic procedures such as an ultrasound scan.

Prevalence ranges from 0.3% as an incidental finding in women undergoing IUD placement to ≥20% in women with a history of postpartum curettage and the number of cases reported has been increasing with the widespread use of hysteroscopy and improvement of imaging tools concentrating on intrauterine pathology.

It is found in 1.5% of women evaluated with a hysterosalpingogram (HSG) for infertility, between 5% and 39% of women with recurrent miscarriage [7].

It may occur in up to 13% of women undergoing a termination of pregnancy during the first trimester, and 30% in women undergoing a dilation and curettage (D and C) after a late spontaneous abortion.

9.3 Etiology and Pathophysiology

The formation of adhesions in an organ that routinely undergoes cyclical change with growth and sloughing is not well understood: intrauterine adhesions (IUAs) are believed to form following a process that damages the basalis layer of the endometrium [8] and the gravid uterus seems particularly susceptible (Table 9.1).

Table 9.1 D&C, dilation and curettage; POC, products of conception; SAB, spontaneous abortion; TOP, termination of pregnancy

Condition	Procedure	Incidence (%)	References
Gravid			
SAB	Suction D&C	15	Gilman et al.
		19	Hooker et al.
First-trimester TOP	Suction D&C	21	Hooker et al.
Retained POC	Hysteroscopic resection	6	Smorgick et al.
		13	Hooker et al.
		19	Barel et al.
	Suction D&C	30	Hooker et al.
Gynecologic			
Septum	Hysteroscopic resection	24	Yu et al.
Fibroids	Hysteroscopic myomectomy	8	Touboul et al.
	Abdominal myomectomy	22	Bhandari et al.

From Salazar CA et al. (2017)

Studying a population of women with confirmation of a normal uterine cavity at baseline, Gilman et al. [9] reported a 15% incidence of IUA formation after suction dilation and curettage by a hysteroscopic follow-up in the ensuing 2–4 months for management of spontaneous abortion (SAB) vs. 1.2% with expectant medical management.

These data are similar to those reported in other papers; a recent systematic meta-analysis reported a similar pooled prevalence of 19% amongst women who suffered a miscarriage and were prospectively assessed by hysteroscopy within 12 months, with over half of the reported cases described as mild adhesive disease [10].

Moreover, the risk and extent of adhesion formation may differ depending on the timing of instrumentation, during early pregnancy versus the postpartum period. Thus up to 21% of women evaluated by hysteroscopy following first-trimester termination of pregnancy shows the formation of a certain degree of IUAs [11].

In one study of women with IUAs, 70% of patients with severe Asherman's had prior instrumentation in the postpartum period, whereas 80–90% of patients with mild Asherman's had procedures performed in the first trimester of pregnancy [12].

Formation of IUA has also been associated with retained products of conception (RPOC) [13]. Amongst women surgically treated for RPOC and evaluated hysteroscopically afterwards, the overall incidence of IUAs varies widely in literature ranging from 6% to 22% [14, 15]. Those treated surgically with dilatation and curettage seem more likely to suffer from IUAs compared to women treated with hysteroscopic resection for RPOC [14]; besides hysteroscopic treatment of RPOC looks to be an opportunity to maximize successful fertility outcomes [16].

IUAs can obviously also develop after gynecologic procedures, such as after resection of uterine septa and leiomyomas.

A large prospective study by Yu et al. [17] evaluating with a second-look hysteroscopy 238 patients previously undergoing hysteroscopic treatment of uterine septa using bipolar energy reported an incidence of IUAs of ≈20%, while newer data regarding incidence of IUA after hysteroscopic myomectomy reveal that the incidence of de novo adhesion formation is less than 10% [14]. This is in contrast to older data reporting rates of adhesion occurring as high as 30–45% [18].

A recent prospective study reported rates of IUA re-formation nearing 22% for abdominal myomectomy procedures as diagnosed by hysteroscopy 3 months after their surgical procedure [19].

Understanding the related molecular mechanisms regulating the pathogenesis of intrauterine adhesions could be the keystone for the prevention of de novo formation and recrudescence and treatment.

It has been reported that postinfectious inflammation and inflammatory factors play important roles in the pathogenesis of AS [2–4, 20–23].

IUAs are in addition caused by infection or injury-related inflammation. It coordinates gene expression and controls the tissue microenvironment especially with cytokines such as TGF-β, TNF-α, IL-1, and IL-18, frequently elevated in intrauterine adhesions, and promoting the pathogenesis of Asherman's syndrome [24].

The nuclear factor-kappaB (NF-κB) transcription factor promotes the expression of intrauterine adhesion inflammatory factors and plays a central role in inflammatory diseases [5, 6, 25–27], and is significantly elevated in endometrial samples from intrauterine adhesion patients compared to normal endometrium controls in human and murine models [24].

However, whether NF-κB promotes the pathogenesis of Asherman's syndrome remains unknown.

9.4 Clinical Presentation

The classic presentation of Asherman's syndrome is an ovulatory patient with onset of secondary amenorrhea after uterine surgery on a gravid uterus and a history of failed provocation of withdrawal bleeding after progesterone administration.

The largest published series to date on the outcomes of hysteroscopic adhesiolysis for Asherman's syndrome reported two-thirds of patients presenting with amenorrhea, while nearly one-third complaining hypomenorrhea (i.e., diminished menstrual flow) [12]. Approximately 3.5% of patients have a primary complaint of cyclic dysmenorrhea. However, menstrual pattern and extent of IUA do not always correlate linearly as a small number of patients (2–5%) may present with regular, painless menses of normal flow and duration despite a severe disease [18].

An ultrasound will demonstrate a hematometra if there are dense lower uterine segment adhesions or cervical adhesions that cause menstrual outflow obstruction; notably, in patients with severe Asherman's syndrome, the increased connective tissue fibrotic and atrophic changes can result in an absence of hematometra despite outflow obstruction [28].

In addition to symptoms of amenorrhea, hypomenorrhea, and cyclical pain, IUA can be associated with infertility and recurrent pregnancy loss.

Synechiae can obstruct the tubal ostia and adhesions may diminish the viable endometrial surface so approximately 7% of patients can present with a primary fertility complaint [12].

IUA can also be asymptomatic, but still may have a negative impact on fertility.

9.5 Workup

In women with suspected Asherman's syndrome, physical examination frequently fails to reveal abnormalities and office ultrasound often fails to detect any aberration.

According to AAGL/ESGE latest practice guidelines (2017) **hysteroscopy** is the most accurate method for diagnosis of IUAs and should be the investigation of choice when available (level of evidence B), as it provides several **advantages**:

1. A real-time view of the cavity
2. Enables accurate description of location and degree of adhesions
3. Precise classification
4. Concurrent treatment of IUAs (*see and treat*)

When hysteroscopy is not available, hysterosalpingography (HSG) and sonohysterography (SHG) with saline infusion sonography (SIS) or gel infusion sonography (GIS) are reasonable alternatives.

Sonohysterography (SHG; also called saline infusion sonography [SIS] or gel infusion sonography [GIS]) was found to be as effective as HSG, with both reported to have a sensitivity of 75% and positive predictive value of 43% for SHG or SIS/GIS and 50% for HSG, compared with hysteroscopy [10, 14]. Three-dimensional SHG has a high specificity of 87% although a lower sensitivity of 70% when compared with the standard hysteroscopy [16].

Magnetic resonance imaging (MRI) for the diagnosis of IUAs is a money- and time-consuming alternative [1, 3, 29–32] and as a matter of fact it is not recommended for clinical practice outside of clinical research studies (Level C) until further research is undertaken.

9.6 Classification System

To date the presence of various classification systems is quite puzzling given the fact that there have been no comparative analyses of the different classifications as the extreme heterogeneity makes appraisal between different series difficult to interpret.

Societies do not endorse any specific system given the deficiencies in each of the following but surely almost all are based on hysteroscopic assessment making this procedure essential since the diagnostic workup.

In the late 1970s, March proposed the first idea for classification based on hysteroscopic findings reporting a series of 66 patients undergoing hysteroscopic evaluation and treatment for Asherman's syndrome.

The idea was to divide those patients using the proportion of cavity interested by adhesions and the characteristics of the findings as follows:

- Severe: >3/4 of uterine cavity is involved; agglutination of walls or thick bands; ostial areas and upper cavity occluded
- Moderate: 1/4 to 3/4 of uterine cavity involved; no agglutination of walls and adhesions only; ostial areas and upper fundus only partially occluded
- Minimal: <1/4 of uterine cavity involved; thin or filmy adhesions; ostial areas and upper fundus minimally involved or clear

Also Professor J. Hamou, the father of modern hysteroscopy, proposed his own way in order to make a reproducible description classifying adhesions as isthmic, marginal, central, or severe according to hysteroscopic assessment.

With the advances in technology and the introduction of new diagnostic tools some authors also included HSG assessment as a combination of hysteroscopic findings or alone when hysteroscopy is not available: hysteroscopy remains a mainstay.

For example European Society of Hysteroscopy [29], American Fertility Society [30], and AAGL grade the clinical findings also accepting a combination of hysteroscopic and HSG findings as a reasonable alternative.

As a matter of fact, the great part of these classifications use hysteroscopic criteria (Table 9.2) and define a scoring system according to the extent of the cavity involvement and/or the severity of the synechiae and/or the extent of occlusion (partial or total).

Table 9.2 Classification of intrauterine adhesions

Source	Summary of classification
March et al.	Adhesions classified as minimal, moderate, or severe based on hysteroscopic assessment of the degree of uterine cavity involvement
Hamou et al.	Adhesions classified as isthmic, marginal, central, or severe according to hysteroscopic assessment
Valle and Sciarra	Adhesions classified as mild, moderate, or severe according to hysteroscopic assessment and extent of occlusion (partial or total) at HSG
European Society of Hysteroscopy	Complex system classifies IUAs as grades I through IV with several subtypes and incorporates a combination of hysteroscopic and HSG findings and clinical symptoms
American Fertility Society	Complex scored system of mild, moderate, or severe IUAs based on the extent of endometrial cavity obliteration, appearance of adhesions, and patient menstrual characteristics based on hysteroscopic or HSG assessment
Donnez and Nisolle	Adhesions classified into six grades on the basis of location, with postoperative pregnancy rate the primary driver. Hysteroscopy or HSG is used for assessment
Nasr et al.	Complex system creates a prognostic score by incorporating menstrual and obstetric history with IUA findings at hysteroscopic assessment

From AAGL practice guidelines on intrauterine adhesions

A commonly used system in the United States is the three-pronged approach provided by the American Society for Reproductive Medicine (ASRM), which defines the severity of intrauterine adhesive disease based on the extent of cavity involvement (<1/3, 1/3 to 2/3, >2/3), the type of adhesion seen (filmy, filmy and dense, dense), as well as the menstrual pattern (normal, hypomenorrhea, amenorrhea). Points are assigned to each finding and the patient is staged from 1 to 3 corresponding to mild, moderate, or severe, based on the total score [33]. The classification system is useful; however, it lacks power in that the staging does not necessarily correlate directly with clinical prognosis [34].

Some other classifications may include other variables such as menstrual and obstetric anamnesis with the findings at the hysteroscopy.

9.7 Treatment

Although a broadly accepted surgical and postoperative flowchart for the management of Asherman's syndrome is difficult to assess, recent American Association of Gynecologic Laparoscopists (AAGL) practice guidelines suggest that high-quality studies and larger case series should be undertaken to provide a more accurate assessment of outcome measures and finally improve the management of this condition.

9.7.1 Hysteroscopic Adhesiolysis

Lysis of intrauterine adhesions under direct hysteroscopic visualization is generally regarded as the mainstay of treatment for Asherman's syndrome; however successful treatment is often difficult to achieve mostly because of the high recurrence rate after hysteroscopic adhesiolysis that is essentially related to the extent and severity of any preexisting lesion and is reported to reach two-thirds in severe cases, more than 20% in moderate cases, and negligible percentages for mild synechiae [35–38].

Hysteroscopic guidance has several advantages:

- Hysteroscopy enables lysis of adhesions under direct visualization and magnification.
- Cavity distension and separation of the uterine walls place bands of fibrosis under tension and this facilitates lysis of adhesions.
- The surgeon can bluntly lyse filmy adhesions (especially central cavity lesions) simply exploiting cavity distension and using the tip of the hysteroscope without any other instrument.
- Operating channels of hysteroscopes can allow various instruments to be used for lysis of firm adhesions: scissors, monopolar energy systems, bipolar energy systems, or neodymium-doped yttrium aluminum garnet [Nd-YAG] laser allows the surgeon bloodless excision also in severe situations.

The basic principle involves beginning adhesiolysis in a caudad to cephalad fashion towards the uterine fundus to enable cavity expansion by the distension media.

The lysis of filmy and central synechiae should be performed first as they are more easily distinguishable; dense synechiae and those of marginal location should be taken down last as they are technically harder to resect and can result in a higher chance of bleeding, complications, and uterine perforation.

The surgeon must remember to lyse the median and avascular portion of the synechiae and both ends will immediately retract into the thickness of the wall leaving behind only two small residual areas on opposing walls of the uterine cavity. The operator usually only needs to move the tip of the hysteroscope to tear down the thinner synechiae while it is not enough to solve the thickest.

In fact, lysis of moderate synechiae often requires the use of hysteroscopic scissors to gradually transect fibrous bridges. The absence of nerve endings or blood vessels in fibrous tissue allows to perform lysis without causing pain or bleeding, which otherwise would impair vision. The major advantage of scissors is their extreme delicacy leaving healthy endometrium untouched. This can decrease the risk for further damage and reduce the risk of recurrence. Additionally, the lack of coagulation while dissecting with scissors can be used to the surgeon's advantage while determining when to stop resection at the uterine fundus. Slight bleeding at the fundus indicates entry into myometrium, a phenomenon that is masked if instruments with coagulation capacity are used.

Severe synechiae may be treated using bipolar electrodes always cutting at the level of the avascular median plane. The use of modern bipolar electrodes, which have a limited surface of exposure to the current, inherently reduces the risk of iatrogenic thermal damage to adjacent healthy endometrium. Another advantage of electrosurgical systems over hysteroscopic scissors is that they cut and also coagulate, thus yielding a better outcome in terms of hemostatic control.

Monopolar instruments require nonelectrolyte distending media like glycine and sorbitol. Excessive absorption of these hypotonic media can lead to hypo-osmolality and hyponatremia, and in extreme cases cerebral edema. The main advantage of this modality is precise and hemostatic resection of disease. The procedure is hence best performed under experienced hands where time management and efficiency of movement in the surgical field are of paramount importance.

Bipolar vaporization of adhesive disease in the uterine cavity using the Versapoint (GYNECARE VERSAPOINT™ Bipolar Electrosurgery System, Johnson & Johnson) instrument has been described. The advantage over monopolar instruments is the fact that these instruments use normal saline isotonic distention media. Even though excessive fluid deficit with normal saline can result in hypervolemia, pulmonary edema, and congestive heart failure, these complications are typically seen at a fluid deficit of >2500 mL and most can be reversed by induced diuresis [39].

Hanstede et al. [40] reported a series of hysteroscopic adhesiolysis performed in 638 patients as a result of a 10-year centralized Asherman's surgery. At the follow-up despite the high proportion of severe cases (60%) a healthy menstrual pattern was restored in 624 (97.8%) within 2 months after initial surgery with an overall success rate (restoration of menses and cavity anatomy) of 95.0% in 1–3 attempts.

From early 1990s onwards most studies reported discordant data with a complete normalization of uterine cavity ranging from 43.7% to 93.3% and restoration of menses ranging from 67.7% to 96% sample sizes. These series are sometimes poorly comparable as they come from a collection of retrospective data and with nonhomogeneous severity of IUAs and consistent biases in population selection [41–50].

Some ancillary techniques have been described to improve the safety in difficult cases of hysteroscopic adhesiolysis (typically with severe occlusive disease) such as the following:

Instillation of methylene blue dye to stain the endometrium and guide the surgeon in between areas of fibrosis as the dye stains endometrium well but uptake into myometrium is not seen.

Transabdominal ultrasound guidance can help to reduce the risk of uterine perforation [23, 28]. The availability and familiarity of sonography to gynecologists make this option easy to implement. Still, uterine perforations in as many as 5% of cases have been reported.

Fluoroscopic guided resection: Fluoroscopic guidance allows the surgeon to view islands of endometrium behind scar tissue in an obliterated uterine cavity. This technique has also been described as an outpatient procedure, though further study is needed [42, 51].

Laparoscopic guided resection: Laparoscopic guidance for severe cases of intrauterine adhesiolysis has been advocated for immediate recognition and treatment of uterine perforation and minimizing extrauterine trauma.

9.7.2 Office Hysteroscopy

Although outpatient hysteroscopy has been gaining popularity rapidly, little data have been reported on the treatment of Asherman's syndrome in this setting.

Outpatient hysteroscopy presents an alternative to traditional hysteroscopy performed in the operating room and offers advantages in terms of reduced anesthetic risks, improved postoperative pain control, faster return to work, and decreased cost [52–60].

Large case series have reported excellent success rates with minimal complications [56–60]. Patients generally report high satisfaction with their procedures performed in an outpatient setting [40] and some have suggested that intrauterine lysis of adhesions can also be performed in this setting [56, 59, 60].

Literature evaluating the feasibility and success rates of treating Asherman's syndrome in outpatient hysteroscopy units shows that surgical treatment may be performed in an office setting with outcomes similar to those in inpatient settings.

Bougie et al. [32] reviewed their data on patients treated in the outpatient hysteroscopy suite at Ottawa Hospital from 2008 to 2013. Patients had regular follow-up clinic appointments after their procedure in order to assess a series of clinical endpoints (regular menses, pregnancy rates). Only 2 out of 19 patients (10%) required hysteroscopic adhesiolysis performed in the main operating room as they required hysteroscopic myomectomy as an adjunct procedure, which could not be performed in the office setting.

The first obvious advantage of the office setting is in regard to the analgesia methods used during each procedure: it is possible to perform even complex procedures with the administration of NSAIDs preoperatively sparing the side effects of intravenous sedation with the use of fentanyl and/or midazolam or more invasive techniques as the paracervical blocks.

Another clear advantage is that we can bring back patients to repeat hysteroscopies until either no adhesions or only mild adhesions are noted. The rationale for this management approach is [32, 61] that repeated adhesiolysis with office hysteroscope allows for the release of thin, filmy adhesions before they have the chance to become dense and/or vascularize and so to prevent recurrence of intrauterine adhesions.

9.8 Postoperative Management

The lack of consensus with regard to the use of postoperative adjuvant treatment to prevent adhesion re-formation and the paucity of well-planned RCT in this area is obvious.

Attention should be focused on reducing the risk of re-formation of IUAs.

Various methods have been described in literature:

- Solid barriers
- Semisolid barriers
- Hormone therapy
- Antibiotics
- Stem cells

Tertiary referral centers which manage a high volume of cases should be encouraged to set up a registry to facilitate the collection of valuable audit data and to conduct RCT to examine the effectiveness, if any, of the various adjuvant treatments in the prevention of recurrence.

9.8.1 Solid Barriers

IUD insertion after hysteroscopic treatment has been described for many years. However, data to support its effectiveness is lacking.

The type of IUD inserted may be important. Copper-containing and T-shaped IUDs cannot be recommended because of their inflammatory provoking properties and small surface area, respectively. Moreover, copper IUD can provoke inflammation and may be counterproductive [62, 63].

The risk of infection after IUD insertion postsurgical resection of IUAs is estimated to be 8% and perforation of the uterus during IUD insertion has been anecdotally reported. The risk of infection when an IUD is introduced into the uterus immediately after adhesiolysis is estimated to be 8%, and perforation of the uterus during IUD insertion has been reported [62–64].

There are few studies comparing IUD use to intrauterine balloon, Foley catheter, and other treatment options such as hormone treatment and barriers like amniotic membranes with low/very-low-quality and underpowered sample sizes, significant heterogeneity, and high risk of biases.

Despite adhesion re-formation being recognized as a biological process that develops over a relatively prolonged period of time, recently the intermittent use of intrauterine balloon dilatation under ultrasound guidance in the postoperative period has been proposed.

9.8.2 Semisolid Barriers

A number of gel adhesion barriers may be suitable for preventing IUAs: auto-cross-linked hyaluronic acid gel, modified hyaluronic acid, fresh amnion, and dry amniotic membranes have been used as an adhesion barrier [76–80, 82].

Data from animal (rabbits) studies are encouraging and report increasing pregnancy rates when hyaluronic acid barriers are used following induced IUAs, but the same fertility data following treatment with a gel barrier in human is still lacking even if auto-cross-linked hyaluronic acid gel shows an advantage when compared to observation alone in preventing re-formation of IUAs at a second-look hysteroscopy.

However a retrospective series found the reduction to be significantly greater in those women using balloon compared with IUD, hyaluronic gel, and observation alone ($p = 0.001$).

Fresh and dry amniotic grafts have been used as an adhesion barrier with fresh amnion showing better results in pilot studies. The complementary use of fresh amnion graft with a Foley catheter has been described.

A recent meta-analysis on the complementary use of amnion graft with an intrauterine catheter showed that amniotic membrane treatment increased the menstrual blood volume after hysteroscopic adhesiolysis with no statistically significant difference in terms of obstetrical outcomes (pregnancy and spontaneous abortion rates) [71–75].

9.8.3 Hormone Therapy

Postoperative treatment with estrogen therapy (e.g., daily conjugated equine estrogen with or without opposing progestin) has not been standardized in terms of dosage, duration, administration route, or combination with progesterone, as data on its cost-effectiveness are scarce (Table 9.3).

Table 9.3 Summary of the various doses of postoperative estrogen therapy used by different investigators after intrauterine adhesiolysis

Type	Daily dose	Duration	Pattern	References
E2	2 mg	2 months	Continuous	Roy et al. (2010) [86]
	4 mg	2 months	Cyclical	Zikopoulos et al. (2004) [77]
		2 months	Continuous	Capella-Allouc, et al. (1999) [35]
		2 months	Continuous	Fernandez et al. (2006) [76]
	4–6 mg	4–10 weeks	Continuous	Myers et al. (2012) [87]
	6 mg	6 weeks	Continuous	Malhotra et al. (2012) [88]
	7.5 mg	2 months	Continuous	March et al. (1976) [27]
	10 mg	3 months	Cyclical	Liu et al. (2016) [89]
	12 mg	3 months	Cyclical	Orhue et al. (2003) [57]
CEE	0.625 mg	14 days	Cyclical	Yasmin et al. (2007) [40]
		1 month	Cyclical	Takai et al. (2015) [90]
		3–4 months	Continuous	Protopapas et al. (1998) [91]
	1.875 mg	60 days	Continuous	Chen et al. (1997) [92]
	2.5 mg	1 month	Cyclical	Amer et al. (2006) [63]
		1 month	Cyclical	Robinson et al. (2008) [38]
		3 weeks	Continuous	Thomson et al. (2007) [41]
	4 mg	2 weeks	Cyclical	Knopman et al. (2005) [93]
		3 months	Cyclical	Salma et al. (2011) [94]
	5 mg	2 months	Cyclical	Pabuccu et al. (2008) [79]
Vaginal micronized E2	6 mg	4 weeks	Cyclical	Dawood et al. (2010) [95]

Adapted from Liu L. et al. 2018

9.8.4 Antibiotics

The concept that infection may be a leading cause of IUA formation has led many surgeons to treat women undergoing surgical lysis of IUAs with preoperative or intraoperative antibiotic therapy, and some continue with postoperative antibiotic therapy in order to reduce the theoretic risk of secondary infection. There are no data regarding the routine use of antibiotics before, during, or after surgical lysis of intrauterine adhesions. Even the American College of Obstetricians and Gynecologists (ACOG) guidelines for antibiotic use in gynecologic procedures do not support antibiotic use for diagnostic or operative hysteroscopy [76].

9.8.5 Stem Cells

Because mesenchymal progenitor cells have various functions that depend on the tissue origin and donor, it is now accepted that human stem cells will be available as cell sources in regenerative medicine. These cells showed their therapeutic contributors in murine models of Asherman's syndrome as they can significantly improve reproductive outcomes.

More recently, the use of stem cell therapy to help regenerate the endometrium holds promise also in humans. Autologous adult BMSC transplantation has been reported to result in regenerating injured endometrium not responding to conventional treatment for AS.

In one report all 16 women treated with uterine intravascular infusions of bone marrow-derived stem cells had return of menses after adhesiolysis, with three spontaneous pregnancies and another seven pregnancies with in vitro fertilization.

As stated by AAGL guidelines it is imperative that well-conducted RCTs are performed to establish the role of stem cells in addition to or independent of surgical treatments before it is made available in our clinical practice.

Our lack of understating of the molecular pathophysiology of intrauterine adhesions has caused a major hurdle in reaching a goal of complete cure mostly in the field of secondary prevention. While surgical management is gaining finesse, on the other hand prevention of recurrences is the perennial object of dispute while the application of contemporary technologies opens unexploited avenues to innovative therapy [77–80].

The joint AAGL and ESGE guidelines also included recommendation for the prevention of adhesion re-formation. The only methods to receive a Level A grade were the solid barriers and semisolid barriers listed above (Table 9.4).

Table 9.4 Guidelines for secondary prevention of intrauterine adhesions

	Statement
1.	The use of an IUD, stent, or catheter appears to reduce the rate of postoperative adhesion re-formation. There are limited data regarding subsequent fertility outcomes when these barriers are used.
2.	The risk of infection appears to be minimal when a solid barrier is used compared with no treatment.
3.	There is no evidence to support or refute the use of preoperative, intraoperative, or postoperative antibiotic therapy in surgical treatment of IUAs.
4.	If an IUD is used postoperatively, it should be inert and have a large surface area such as a Lippes loop. Intrauterine devices that contain progestin or copper should not be used after surgical division of IUAs.
5.	Semisolid barriers such as hyaluronic acid and auto-cross-linked hyaluronic acid gel reduce adhesion re-formation. At this time, their effect on post-treatment pregnancy rates is unknown.
6.	Following hysteroscopic directed adhesiolysis, postoperative hormone treatment using estrogen, with or without progestin, may reduce recurrence of IUAs.
7.	The role of medications designed as adjuvants to improve vascular flow to the endometrium has not been established. Consequently, they should not be used outside of rigorous research protocols.
8.	Stem cell treatment may ultimately provide an effective adjuvant approach to the treatment of Asherman's syndrome; however, evidence is very limited and this treatment should not be offered outside of rigorous research protocols.

9.9 Prognosis

Even if it is not a life-threatening condition, AS surely affects quality of life as the reproductive outcome after hysteroscopic adhesiolysis in women with AS has been reported in a number of studies and the reported pregnancy rate after hysteroscopic management ranges from 10.5% to 100%.

The results are variable due to a number of biases: firstly, the confounding variables including the age of the subjects, the severity of the IUA, the duration of follow-up, and the coexistence of any other infertility factors and then many of the reported studies that consisted of small numbers with a relatively wide confidence interval.

Recently a systematic review of literature based on 54 studies including nearly 4600 women found a certain relationship between the severity of adhesion and pregnancy rate: amongst women with mild, moderate, and severe IUA, the median pregnancy rates were 69.1%, 61.3%, and 44.3%, respectively, and the pregnant rate was significantly decreased in severe adhesion group when compared to mild adhesion group.

Moreover, pregnancy occurring in women after surgical treatment of IUA was associated with a number of obstetric complications, including ectopic pregnancy, cervical incompetence, midtrimester loss, placenta previa, placenta abruption, premature rupture of membrane, placenta accrete syndrome, neonatal death, and stillbirth when compared with general population and this suggests that conceiving after surgical treatment of AS requires increased surveillance during their pregnancy.

Women should be offered an earlier ultrasound examination to verify the location of the pregnancy; the fallopian tube is the most common location of ectopic pregnancy (~95%); however, implantation in the abdomen (<1%), cervix (1%), ovary (1–3%), and caesarean scar (1–3%) can occur [11, 74].

Key Points

1. Lysis of intrauterine adhesions under direct hysteroscopic visualization is generally regarded as the mainstay of treatment for Asherman's syndrome.
2. Hysteroscopic lysis can be done using scissors, monopolar energy systems, bipolar energy systems, or neodymium-doped yttrium aluminum garnet [Nd-YAG] laser.
3. In experienced hands, vaginoscopy—no-speculum hysteroscopy—prevents trauma and can help in severe cases of IUA.
4. Mechanical separation of IUA using scissors is the most accessible means of adhesiolysis.
5. Myometrial scoring technique has been effective for the creation of a uterine cavity in women with severe IUAs having very narrow or obliterated cavity.
6. Assisted or ancillary or guided techniques have been described to improve the safety in difficult and severe occlusive disease.

References

1. Fritsch H. Ein Fall von voelligem Schwund der Gebarmutterhoehle nach Auskratzung. Zentralbl Gynakol. 1894;18:1337–9.
2. Stamer S. Partial and total atresia of the uterus after excochleation. Acta Obstet Gynecol Scand. 1946;26:263–97.
3. Asherman JG. Amenorrhoea traumatica (atretica). J Obstet Gynaecol Br Emp. 1948;55:23–30.
4. Asherman JG. Traumatic intrauterine adhesions. J Obstet Gynaecol Br Emp. 1950;57:892–6.
5. Asherman JG. Traumatic intrauterine adhesions and their effects on fertility. Int J Fertil. 1957;2:49–54.
6. Asherman JG. Les adherences intrauterines. Rev Fr Gynecol Obstet. 1961;56:311.
7. Smikle C. Shailesh Khetarpal Asherman Syndrome. Treasure Island, FL: StatPearls Publishing LLC; 2019.
8. Dalton VK, Saunders NA, Harris LH, Williams JA, Lebovic DI. Intrauterine adhesions after manual vacuum aspiration for early pregnancy failure. Fertil Steril. 2006;85:1823.e1e3.
9. Gilman AR, Dewar KM, Rhone SA, Fluker MR. Intrauterine adhesions following miscarriage: look and learn. J Obstet Gynaecol Can. 2016;38:453–7. A well designed retrospective study evaluating the incidence of IUA after management of miscarriage in a cohort of patients with a documented normal cavity.
10. Hooker AB, Lemmers M, Thurkow AL, et al. Systematic review and meta-analysis of intrauterine adhesions after miscarriage: prevalence, risk factors and long-term reproductive outcome. Hum Reprod Update. 2014;20:262–78.
11. Hooker A, Fraenk D, Brolmann H, Huirne J. Prevalence of intrauterine adhesions after termination of pregnancy: a systematic review. Eur J Contract Reprod Health Care. 2016;21:329–35.
12. Hanstede MMF, van der Meij E, Goedemans L, Emanuel MH. Results of centralized Asherman surgery, 2003–2013. Fertil Steril. 2015;104:1561–8. (The largest published series to date on the outcomes of hysteroscopic adhesiolysis for Asherman's syndrome.)
13. Hooker AB, Muller LT, Paternotte E, Thurkow AL. Immediate and long-term complications of delayed surgical management in the postpartum period: a retrospective analysis. J Matern-Fetal Neonatal Med. 2015;28:1884–9.
14. Hooker AB, Aydin H, Brolmann HAM, Huirne JAF. Long-term complications and reproductive outcome after the management of retained products of conception: a systematic review. Fertil Steril. 2016;105:156–64.
15. Barel O, Krakov A, Pansky M, et al. Intrauterine adhesions after hysteroscopic treatment for retained products of conception: what are the risk factors? Fertil Steril. 2015;103:775–9.
16. Sonnier L, Torre A, Broux P, et al. Evaluation of fertility after operative hysteroscopy to remove retained products of conception. Eur J Obstet Gynecol Reprod Biol. 2017;211:98–102.
17. Yu X, Yuhan L, Dongmei S, et al. The incidence of postoperative adhesion following transection of uterine septum: a cohort study comparing three different adjuvant therapies. Eur J Obstet Gynecol Reprod Biol. 2016;201:61–4.
18. March CM. Management of Asherman's syndrome. Reprod BioMed Online. 2011;23:63–76.
19. Bhandari S, Ganguly I, Agarwal P, et al. Effect of myomectomy on endometrial cavity: a prospective study of 51 cases. J Hum Reprod Sci. 2016;9:107–11.
20. Li Q, Verma IM. NF-kappaB regulation in the immune system. Nat Rev Immunol. 2002;2:725–34. https://doi.org/10.1038/nri910.
21. Liang Y, Zhou Y, Shen P. NF-kappaB and its regulation on the immune system. Cell Mol Immunol. 2004;1:343–50.
22. Yimam M, Lee YC, Moore B, Jiao P, Hong M, Nam JB, Kim MR, Hyun EJ, Chu M, Brownell L, Jia Q. Analgesic and anti-inflammatory effects of UP1304, a botanical composite containing standardized extracts of Curcuma longa and Morus alba. J Integr Med. 2016;14:60–8.
23. Yu D, Wong YM, Cheong Y, Xia E, Li TC. Asherman syndrome—one century later. Fertil Steril. 2008;89(4):759–79.

24. Wang X, Ma N, Sun Q, Huang C, Liu Y, Luo X. Elevated NF-κB signaling in Asherman syndrome patients and animal models. Oncotarget. 2017;8(9):15399–406.
25. Tsui KH, Lin L, Te Cheng JT, Teng SW, Wang PH. Comprehensive treatment for infertile women with severe Asherman syndrome. Taiwan J Obstet Gynecol. 2014;53:372–5.
26. Vesce F, Jorizzo G, Bianciotto A, Gotti G. Use of the copper intrauterine device in the management of secondary amenorrhea. Fertil Steril. 2000;73:162–5.
27. March CM, Israel R. Gestational outcomes following hysteroscopic lysis of adhesions. Fertil Steril. 1981;36:455–9.
28. Deans R, Abbott J. Review of intrauterine adhesions. J Minim Invasive Gynecol. 2010;17:555–69.
29. Wamsteker K, De Blok SJ. Diagnostic hysteroscopy: technique and documentation. In: Sutton C, Diamon M, editors. Endoscopic surgery for gynecologists. New York: Lippincott Williams & Wilkins Publishers; 1995. p. 263–76.
30. AAGL Practice Report. Practice Guidelines on Intrauterine Adhesions Developed in Collaboration With the European Society of Gynaecological Endoscopy (ESGE). J Minim Invasive Gynecol. 2017;24(5):695–705. https://doi.org/10.1016/j.jmig.2016.11.008.
31. Khan Z, Goldberg JM. Hysteroscopic management of Asherman's syndrome: special issue report on uterine surgery. J Minim Invasive Gynecol. 2018;25(2):218–28. https://doi.org/10.1016/j.jmig.2017.09.020.
32. Bougie O, Lortie K, Shenassa H, Chen I, Singh SS. Treatment of Asherman's syndrome in an outpatient hysteroscopy setting. J Minim Invasive Gynecol. 2015;22(3):446–50.
33. The American Fertility Society. Classifications of adnexal adhesions, distal tubal occlusion, tubal occlusion secondary to tubal ligation, tubal pregnancies, Mullerian anomalies and intrauterine adhesions. Fertil Steril. 1988;49:944–55.
34. Amin TN, Saridogan E, Jurkovic D. Ultrasound and intrauterine adhesions: a novel structured approach to diagnosis and management. Ultrasound Obstet Gynecol. 2015;46:131–9.
35. Capella-Allouc S, Morsad F, Rongieres-Bertrand C, Taylor S, Fernandez H. Hysteroscopic treatment of severe Asherman's syndrome and subsequent fertility. Hum Reprod. 1999;14:1230–3.
36. Preutthipan S, Linasmita V. A prospective comparative study between hysterosalpingography and hysteroscopy in the detection of intrauterine pathology in patients with infertility. J Obstet Gynaecol Res. 2003;29:33–7.
37. Siegler A, Valle R. Therapeutic hysteroscopic procedures. Fertil Steril. 1988;50:685–701.
38. Robinson JK, Swedarsky Colimon LM, Isaacson KB. Postoperative adhesiolysis therapy for intrauterine adhesions (Asherman's syndrome). Fertil Steril. 2008;90:409–14.
39. Zikopoulos K. Live delivery rates in subfertile women with Asherman's syndrome after hysteroscopic adhesiolysis using the resectoscope or the Versapoint system. Reprod BioMed Online. 2004;8:720–5.
40. Hanstede MMF, van der Meij E, Goedemans L, Emanuel MH. Results of centralized Asherman surgery, 2003–2013. Fertil Steril. 2015;104(6):1561-8.e1.
41. Yasmin H, Nasir A, Noorani KJ. Hysteroscopic management of Asherman's syndrome. J Pak Med Assoc. 2007;57:553–5.
42. Thomson AJ, Abbott JA, Kingston A, Lenart M, Vancaillie TG. Fluoroscopically guided synechiolysis for patients with Asherman's syndrome: menstrual and fertility outcomes. Fertil Steril. 2007;87:405–10.
43. Al-Inany H. Intrauterine adhesions. An update. Acta Obstet Gynecol Scand. 2001;80:986–93.
44. Schenker JG, Margalioth EJ. Intrauterine adhesions: an updated appraisal. Fertil Steril. 1982;37:593–610.
45. Polishuk WZ, Siew FP, Gordon R, Lebenshart P. Vascular changes in traumatic amenorrhea and hypomenorrhea. Int J Fertil. 1977;22:189–92.
46. Liu F, Zhu ZJ, Li P, He YL. Creation of a female rabbit model for intrauterine adhesions using mechanical and infectious injury. J Surg Res. 2013;183:296–303.
47. Tao Z, Duan H. Expression of adhesion-related cytokines in the uterine fluid after transcervical resection of adhesion. Zhonghua Fu Chan Ke Za Zhi. 2012;47:734–7.

48. Sillem M, Prifti S, Monga B, Arslic T, Runnebaum B. Integrin-mediated adhesion of uterine endometrial cells from endometriosis patients to extracellular matrix proteins is enhanced by tumor necrosis factor alpha (TNF alpha) and interleukin-1 (IL-1). Eur J Obstet Gynecol Reprod Biol. 1999;87:123–7.
49. Lawrence T. The nuclear factor NF-kappaB pathway in inflammation. Cold Spring Harb Perspect Biol. 2009;1:a001651. https://doi.org/10.1101/cshperspect.a001651.
50. Tak PP, Firestein GS. NF-kappaB: a key role in inflammatory diseases. J Clin Invest. 2001;107:7–11. https://doi.org/10.1172/JCI11830.
51. Broome JD, Vancaillie TG. Fluoroscopically guided hysteroscopic division of adhesions in severe Asherman syndrome. Obstet Gynecol. 1999;93:1041–3.
52. Bettocchi S, Ceci O, Nappi L, et al. Operative office hysteroscopy without anesthesia: Analysis of 4863 cases performed with mechanical instruments. J Am Assoc Gynecol Laparosc. 2004;11:59–61.
53. Cicinelli E, Parisi C, Galantino P, Pinto V, Barba B, Schonauer S. Reliability, feasibility, and safety of minihysteroscopy with a vaginoscopic approach: experience with 6,000 cases. Fertil Steril. 2003;80:199–202.
54. Van Kerkvoorde TC, Veersema S, Timmermans A. Long-term complications of office hysteroscopy: analysis of 1028 cases. J Minim Invasive Gynecol. 2012;19:494–7.
55. Bettocchi S, Nappi L, Ceci O, Selvaggi L. What does 'diagnostic hysteroscopy' mean today? The role of the new techniques. Curr Opin Obstet Gynecol. 2003;15:303–8.
56. Di Spiezio Sardo A, Bettocchi S, Spinelli M, et al. Review of new office-based hysteroscopic procedures 2003–2009. J Minim Invasive Gynecol. 2010;17:436–48.
57. Bettocchi S, Bramante S, Bifulco G, Spinelli M, Ceci O, Fascilla FD, Di Spiezio Sardo A. Challenging the cervix: strategies to overcome the anatomic impediments to hysteroscopy: analysis of 31,052 office hysteroscopies. Fertil Steril. 2016;105(5):e16–7. https://doi.org/10.1016/j.fertnstert.2016.01.030.
58. Di Spiezio Sardo A, Taylor A, Tsirkas P, Mastrogamvrakis G, Sharma M, Magos A. Hysteroscopy: a technique for all? Analysis of 5,000 outpatient hysteroscopies. Fertil Steril. 2008;89(2):438–43.
59. Fedele L, Vercellini P, Viezzoli T, Ricciardiello O, Zamberletti D. Intrauterine adhesions: current diagnostic and therapeutic trends. Acta Eur Fertil. 1986;17:31–7.
60. Pace S, Stentella P, Catania R, Palazzetti PL, Frega A. Endoscopic treatment of intrauterine adhesion. Clin Exp Obstet Gynecol. 2003;30:26–8.
61. Bougie O, Wang V, Lortie K, Shenassa H, Singh SS. High patient satisfaction with office hysteroscopy using tailored analgesia protocols. J Gynecol Surg. 2014;30:100–4.
62. Orhue AA, Aziken ME, Igbefoh JO. A comparison of two adjunctive treatments for intrauterine adhesions following lysis. Int J Gynaecol Obstet. 2003;82:49–56.
63. Lin XN, Zhou F, Wei ML, et al. Randomized, controlled trial comparing the efficacy of intrauterine balloon and intrauterine contraceptive device in the prevention of adhesion reformation after hysteroscopic adhesiolysis. Fertil Steril. 2015;104:235–40.
64. Sanfilippo JS, Fitzgerald MR, Badawy SZ, Nussbaum ML, Yussman MA. Asherman's syndrome. A comparison of therapeutic methods. J Reprod Med. 1982;27:328–30.
65. Pabuccu R, Onalan G, Kaya C, Selam B, Ceyhan T, Ornek T, Kuzudisli E. Efficiency and pregnancy outcome of serial intrauterine device-guided hysteroscopic adhesiolysis of intrauterine synechiae. Fertil Steril. 2008;90:1973–7.
66. Tsapanos VS, Stathopoulou LP, Papathanassopoulou VS, Tzingounis VA. The role of Seprafilm bioresorbable membrane in the prevention and therapy of endometrial synechiae. J Biomed Mater Res. 2002;63:10–4.
67. Hooker AB, de Leeuw R, van de Ven PM, et al. Prevalence of intrauterine adhesions after the application of hyaluronic acid gel after dilatation and curettage in women with at least one previous curettage: short-term outcomes of a multicenter, prospective randomized controlled trial. Fertil Steril. 2017;107:1223–31.
68. Farhi J, Bar-Hava I, Homburg R, Dicker D, Ben-Rafael Z. Induced regeneration of endometrium following curettage for abortion: a comparative study. Hum Reprod. 1993;8:1143–4.

69. Acunzo G, Guida M, Pellicano M, et al. Effectiveness of auto-crosslinked hyaluronic acid gel in the prevention of intrauterine adhesions after hysteroscopic adhesiolysis: a prospective, randomized, controlled study. Hum Reprod. 2003;18:1918–21.
70. Shi X, Saravelos SH, Zhou Q, Huang X, Xia E, Li TC. Prevention of postoperative adhesion reformation by intermittent intrauterine balloon therapy: a randomised controlled trial. BJOG. 2019;126(10):1259–66.
71. Huberlant S, Fernandez H, Vieille P, Khrouf M, Ulrich D, de Tayrac R, Letouzey V. Application of a hyaluronic acid gel after intrauterine surgery may improve spontaneous fertility: a randomized controlled trial in New Zealand White rabbits. PLoS One. 2015;10:e0125610.
72. Lin X, Wei M, Li TC, Huang Q, Huang D, Zhou F, Zhang S. A comparison of intrauterine balloon, intrauterine contraceptive device and hyaluronic acid gel in the prevention of adhesion reformation following hysteroscopic surgery for Asherman syndrome: a cohort study. Eur J Obstet Gynecol Reprod Biol. 2013;170:512–6.
73. Amer MI, Abd-El-Maeboud KH, Abdelfatah I, Salama FA, Abdallah AS. Human amnion as a temporary biologic barrier after hysteroscopic lysis of severe intrauterine adhesions: pilot study. J Minim Invasive Gynecol. 2010;17:605–11.
74. Amer MI, Abd-El-Maeboud KH. Amnion graft following hysteroscopic lysis of intrauterine adhesions. J Obstet Gynaecol Res. 2006;32:559–66.
75. Zheng F, Zhu B, Liu Y, Wang R, Cui Y. Meta-analysis of the use of amniotic membrane to prevent recurrence of intrauterine adhesion after hysteroscopic adhesiolysis. Int J Gynaecol Obstet. 2018;143(2):145–9.
76. Bulletins ACoP. ACOG Practice Bulletin No. 74. Antibiotic prophylaxis for gynecologic procedures. Obstet Gynecol. 2006;108:225–34.
77. Jun SM, Park M, Lee JY, Jung S, Lee JE, Shim SH, Song H, Lee DR. Single cell-derived clonally expanded mesenchymal progenitor cells from somatic cell nuclear transfer-derived pluripotent stem cells ameliorate the endometrial function in the uterus of a murine model with Asherman's syndrome. Cell Prolif. 2019;52(3):e12597.
78. Gao L, Huang Z, Lin H, Tian Y, Li P, Lin S. Bone marrow mesenchymal stem cells (BMSCs) restore functional endometrium in the rat model for severe Asherman syndrome. Reprod Sci. 2019;26(3):436–44. https://doi.org/10.1177/1933719118799201.
79. Nagori CB, Panchal SY, Patel H. Endometrial regeneration using autologous adult stem cells followed by conception by in vitro fertilization in a patient of severe Asherman's syndrome. J Hum Reprod Sci. 2011;4(1):43–8.
80. Santamaria X, Cabanillas S, Cervello I, et al. Autologous cell therapy with CD133+ bone marrow-derived stem cells for refractory Asherman's syndrome and endometrial atrophy: a pilot cohort study. Hum Reprod. 2016;31:1087–96.
81. Salazar CA, Isaacson K, Morris S. A comprehensive review of Asherman's syndrome: causes, symptoms and treatment options. Curr Opin Obstet Gynecol. 2017;29(4):249–56.
82. Valle RF, Sciarra JJ. Intrauterine adhesions: hysteroscopic diagnosis, classification, treatment, and reproductive outcome. Am J Obstet Gynecol. 1988;158:1459–70.
83. Fernandez H, Al Najjar F, Chauvenaud-Lambling A, Frydman R, Gervaise A. Fertility after treatment of Asherman's syndrome stage 3 and 4. J Minim Invasive Gynecol. 2006;13:398–402.
84. March CM, Israel R, March AD. Hysteroscopic management of intrauterine adhesions. Am J Obstet Gynecol. 1978;130:653–7.
85. Kodaman PH, Arici A. Intra-uterine adhesions and fertility outcome: how to optimize success? Curr Opin Obstet Gynecol. 2007;19:207–14.
86. Roy KK, Negi N, Subbaiah M, Kumar S, Sharma JB, Singh N. Effectiveness of estrogen in the prevention of intrauterine adhesions after hysteroscopic septal resection: a prospective, randomized study. J Obstet Gynaecol Res. 2014;40(4):1085–8. https://doi.org/10.1111/jog.12297. Epub 2014. Feb 26. PMID: 24612233.
87. Myers EM, Hurst BS. Comprehensive management of severe Asherman syndrome and amenorrhea. Fertil Steril. 2012;97(1):160–4. https://doi.org/10.1016/j.fertnstert.2011.10.036. Epub 2011 Nov 17. PMID: 22100167.

88. Malhotra N, Bahadur A, Kalaivani M, Mittal S. Changes in endometrial receptivity in women with Asherman's syndrome undergoing hysteroscopic adhesiolysis. Arch Gynecol Obstet. 2012;286(2):525–30. https://doi.org/10.1007/s00404-012-2336-0. Epub 2012. PMID: 22535194.
89. Liu AZ, Zhao HG, Gao Y, Liu M, Guo BZ. Effectiveness of estrogen treatment before transcervical resection of adhesions on moderate and severe uterine adhesion patients. Gynecol Endocrinol. 2016;32(9):737–40. https://doi.org/10.3109/09513590.2016.1160375. Epub 2016 Mar 16. PMID: 26982384.
90. Takai IU, Kwayabura AS, Ugwa EA, Idrissa A, Obed JY, Bukar M. A 10-year Review of the Clinical Presentation and Treatment Outcome of Asherman's Syndrome at a Center with Limited Resources. Ann Med Health Sci Res. 2015;5(6):442–6. https://doi.org/10.4103/2141-9248.177984. PMID: 27057384; PMCID: PMC4804657.
91. Protopapas A, Shushan A, Magos A. Myometrial scoring: a new technique for the management of severe Asherman's syndrome. Fertil Steril. 1998;69(5):860–4. https://doi.org/10.1016/s0015-0282(98)00036-3. PMID: 9591493.
92. Chen FP, Soong YK, Hui YL. Successful treatment of severe uterine synechiae with transcervical resectoscopy combined with laminaria tent. Hum Reprod. 1997;12(5):943–7. https://doi.org/10.1093/humrep/12.5.943. PMID: 9194644.
93. Knopman J, Copperman AB. Value of 3D ultrasound in the management of suspected Asherman's syndrome. J Reprod Med. 2007;52(11):1016–22. PMID: 18161399.
94. Salma, U., Xu, D., & Sheikh, M. (1). Diagnosis and treatment of intrauterine adhesions. Bangladesh Journal of Medical Science. 10(2):72–82.
95. Dawood A, Al-Talib A, Tulandi T. Predisposing factors and treatment outcome of different stages of intrauterine adhesions. J Obstet Gynaecol Can. 2010;32(8):767–70. https://doi.org/10.1016/s1701-2163(16)34618-7. PMID: 21050509.

Role of Assisted Operative Hysteroscopy in Asherman's Management

10

Jude E. Okohue

Asherman's syndrome describes the occurrence of intrauterine adhesions in association with symptoms such as menstrual irregularities, recurrent pregnancy loss, and infertility. It is most often preceded by pregnancy-related procedures such as curettage of a pregnant or recently pregnant uterus. Hysteroscopy remains the gold standard in the treatment of Asherman's syndrome. There is limited evidence regarding the ideal treatment modality and randomized controlled trials are needed to determine the optimum modality for prevention of recurrence.

10.1 Introduction

It was Heinrich Fritsch who in 1894 described and published the first case of intrauterine adhesions (IUAs). It however took another 54 years for Joseph Asherman to fully characterize the condition. Asherman initially reported his findings in 29 women who presented with amenorrhea and associated cervical stenosis. He later confirmed intrauterine adhesions involving the endometrial cavity following hysterosalpingography. While intrauterine adhesions describe the occurrence of scar tissues within the uterine cavity, the term Asherman's syndrome is used when IUAs are associated with symptoms such as menstrual irregularities, recurrent pregnancy loss, and infertility.

Intrauterine adhesions and Asherman's syndrome are commonly used interchangeably; some are of the opinion that Asherman's syndrome should only be used when the cause of the IUA is pregnancy related.

J. E. Okohue (✉)
Gynescope Specialist Hospital, Port Harcourt, Rivers, Nigeria

R. Manchanda (ed.), *Intra Uterine Adhesions*,
https://doi.org/10.1007/978-981-33-4145-6_10

10.1.1 Pathophysiology

There are limited data regarding the pathophysiology of Asherman's syndrome. There are possible roles for adhesion-related cytokines such as b-fibroblast growth factor, platelet-derived growth factor, and transforming growth factor type 1 [1].

Schenker and Margalioth [2] found the highest association of Asherman's syndrome among women who had curettage after a miscarriage. The highest incidence of IUA was found in a study, when the curettage was performed between the second and fourth postpartum week [3].

Hysteroscopic division of intrauterine adhesions may be technically difficult, especially if the adhesions are dense. It carries a significant risk of perforation of the uterus, especially during the dilatation of the cervical channel and introduction of the hysteroscope. The introduction of the dilator and hysteroscope must be guided carefully by one of the methods described here to avoid perforation because perforation at this early stage would preclude satisfactory completion of the hysteroscopy. The efficiency and safety of hysteroscopic surgery for Asherman's syndrome may be improved if the procedure is guided by one of the following methods described in this chapter.

10.1.2 Management

Not all cases of IUA require treatment. Historically, IUAs were managed by blind adhesiolysis. The management of severe Asherman's syndrome is still rather challenging despite the widespread use of diagnostic and operative hysteroscopy. In 1978, Sugimoto [4] described the findings of IUA in 192 patients undergoing diagnostic hysteroscopy. Out of these, 143 recovered previous menstrual flow. He however voiced out his frustration at treating severe IUA. Some level of frustration still persists today!

Hysteroscopy remains the gold standard in the diagnosis and treatment of Asherman's syndrome. Hysteroscopy not only allows for the direct visualization of the IUA, but also helps in the classification of the condition.

10.1.3 Aims of Hysteroscopy

1. Restoration of the anatomical shape and capacity of the uterine cavity
2. Restoration of menstruation
3. Restoration of fertility, by ensuring the normal continuity between the tubal ostia, endometrial cavity, and cervical canal

10.1.4 Technique of Hysteroscopic Adhesiolysis

Asherman's syndrome, although a rare condition, was the commonest indication for operative hysteroscopy, in a study performed in an environment with highly

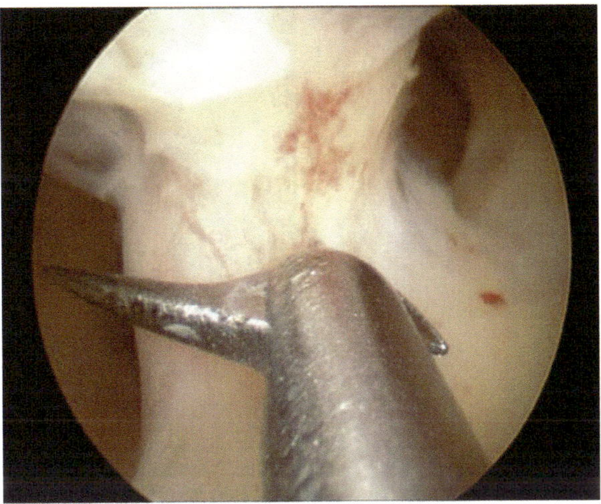

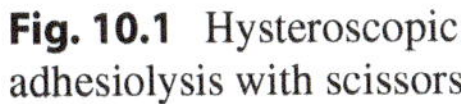

Fig. 10.1 Hysteroscopic adhesiolysis with scissors

restrictive abortion laws [5]. It is the procedure considered to be the most difficult of all the hysteroscopic procedures and therefore it is associated with the greatest risk of complications, especially uterine perforation (ESGE and AAGL standards and guidelines).

The following question has always arisen: Whether to use hysteroscopic scissors or electrocautery (Figs. 10.1 and 10.2) for adhesiolysis?

There are presently no comparative studies and therefore most hysteroscopists tend to use whichever they are conversant with. The author, in his almost two decades' experience with operative hysteroscopy, working in an environment with highly restrictive abortion laws and considerably high unsafe abortion rates, has not had cause to use energy (electrocautery) for hysteroscopic adhesiolysis.

Mild-to-moderate cases might be managed on an outpatient basis without any need for anesthesia, while severe cases are generally managed under general or regional anesthesia.

10.1.5 Important Differences Between Hysteroscopic Scissors and Electrocautery

1. Cautery is more likely to cause damage to the endometrium compared with scissors [6].
2. Following inadvertent perforation of the uterus, significant bowel or urinary bladder injury is more likely with cautery.
3. The use of the resectoscope is likely to be more expensive compared with scissors.
4. The resectoscope would more likely require cervical dilatation compared with the scissors.
5. The use of cautery is however associated with better ability to secure hemostasis.

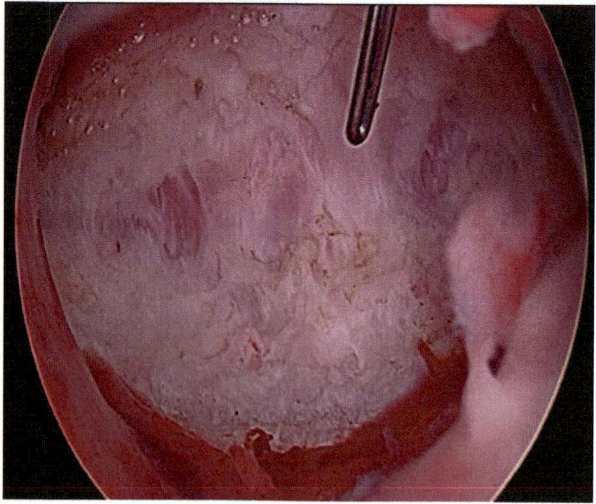

Fig. 10.2 Hysteroscopic adhesiolysis with cautery. Courtesy of Prof. N. Malhotra

Laser vaporization using Nd-YAG (neodymium-doped yttrium aluminum garnet) and KTP (potassium titanyl phosphate) is generally not widespread on account of its higher cost and damage to the endometrial cavity.

If electrocautery is chosen for hysteroscopic adhesiolysis, monopolar and bipolar energy can be used. While both provide satisfactory results, bipolar cautery has the advantage that it is used with electrolyte-containing fluid such as normal saline for uterine distension. Over 2 L of fluid deficit is required for normal saline to cause any serious issue with fluid overload. On the other hand, monopolar energy requires nonelectrolyte-containing fluids such as glycine. A deficit greater than 1 L of glycine might lead to serious complications of fluid overload.

In performing hysteroscopic adhesiolysis, it is important to note that more centrally placed adhesions are less vascularized and less dense, compared with adhesions that are more laterally placed. It is therefore good practice to commence with the more centrally placed adhesions working towards the lateral walls. Distal adhesions are also often dealt with first before the proximal or fundal adhesions.

In case of mild adhesions as shown in Fig. 10.3 (European Society of Hysteroscopy classification, grade 1), the pressure from the distension fluid might be enough to separate the adhesions. Some adhesions are easily separated with the use of the tip of the hysteroscope and sheath. Figure 10.4a–c shows other forms of IUA.

During surgery, it is prudent to be gentle at all times while ensuring a clear operating field, especially with the use of cautery, to prevent uterine perforation. Care must be taken to search for possible routes into the uterine cavity.

When the uterine cavity is completely obliterated due to severe disease (Fig. 10.5), it poses a major challenge. Occasionally, it might be difficult introducing the hysteroscope and sheaths in order to perform an adhesiolysis.

Various techniques have been described with the aim of re-establishing the anatomy of the endometrial cavity. These include the myometrial scoring technique in

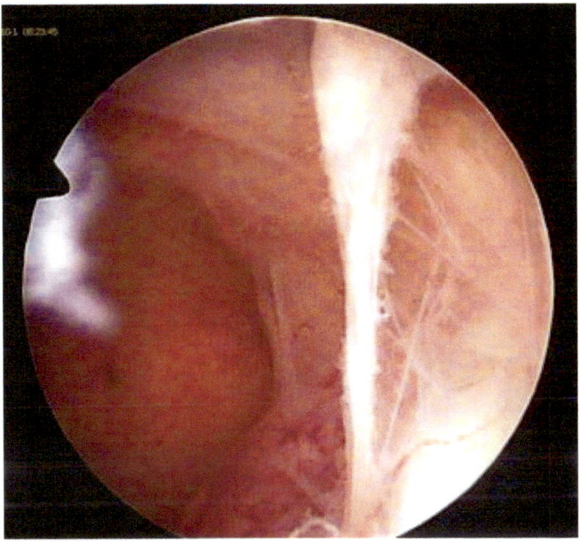

Fig. 10.3 Mild intrauterine adhesions with associated submucous fibroid

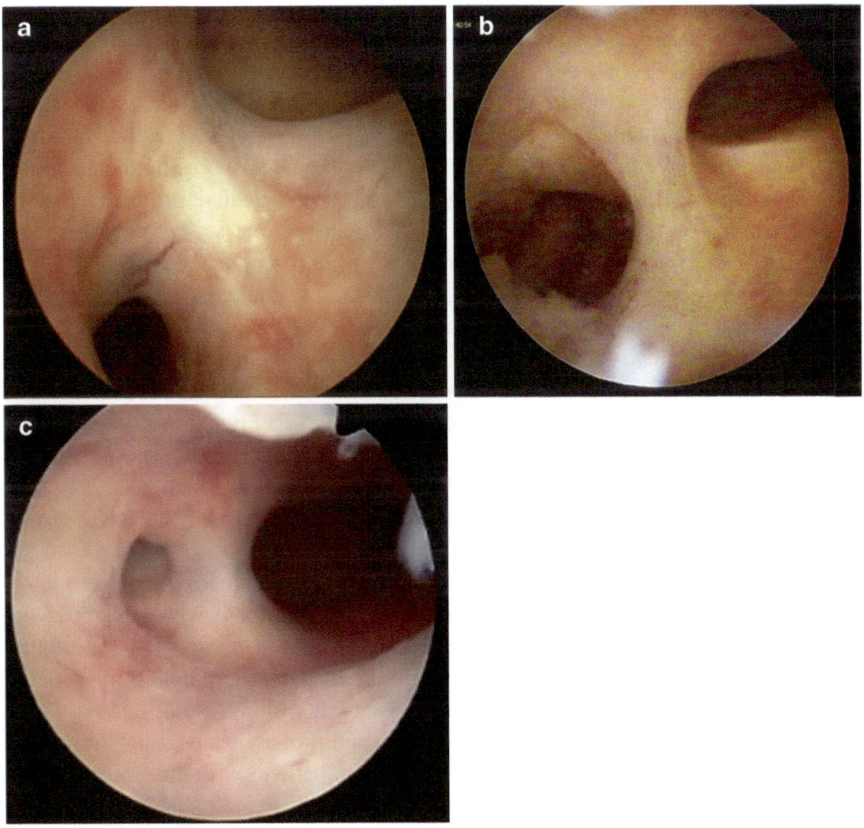

Fig. 10.4 (**a**, **b**) Hysteroscopy showing dense adhesions involving 2/3rd cavity. (**c**) Dense adhesions involving >2/3rd cavity

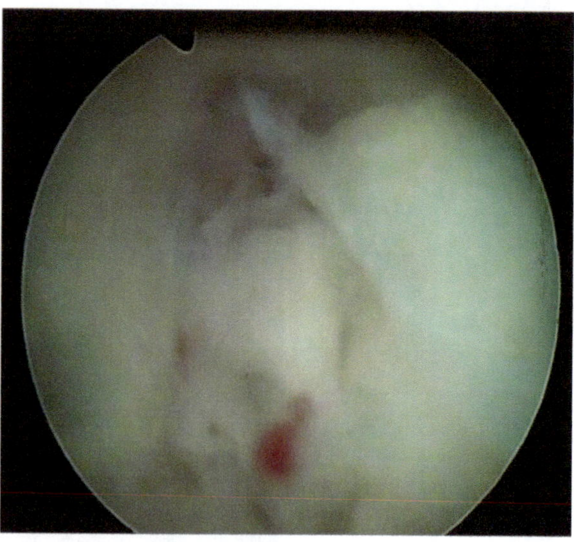

Fig. 10.5 Adhesions involving the entire cavity

which six to eight, 4 mm deep incisions are made within the uterine cavity, from the fundus to the isthmus, using a Collings knife electrode. The cervical os is dilated up to Hegar's size 12–18 in order to perform the procedure.

Another reported technique involved the use of a sharp needle called the Tuohy needle. The needle, which is a 16-gauge type, is introduced alongside a 5 mm hysteroscope. The surgeon then probes areas beyond the adhesion using the needle. A contrast medium, Ultravist 76.9%, is injected via the needle under fluoroscopic and hysteroscopic control. Hidden pockets of endometrium are seen radiographically and subsequent division of the adhesions using hysteroscopic scissors ensures that a passageway is created. All the patients in this series required more than one procedure (one had six procedures performed). While all the 55 women treated with this technique regained normal menstrual function, the authors were silent about the fertility outcome.

A third technique involved the introduction of two 13 French Pratt cones under laparoscopic guidance, via the cervix and towards the ipsilateral tubal cornu, thereby creating a central residual septum. The septum was then hysteroscopically cut with scissors, thus creating a cavity. The technique is not recommended due to the associated morbidities.

In a case series involving seven patients, one or two laminaria tents were introduced to dilate the cervix. After 24 hours of insertion, these were replaced with three or four laminaria tents, now inserted up to the fundus and left for another 24 hours. The procedure was concluded with the hysteroscopic adhesiolysis under laparoscopic guidance and an intrauterine device left within the uterine cavity. The patients were subsequently placed on estrogen and progesterone preparations. The authors reported normal menstrual flow in all seven patients with three pregnancies, including a miscarriage and two live births [7].

10.2 Role of Assisted Adhesiolysis

Modalities such as ultrasound scan, laparoscopy, and fluoroscopy have been proposed for the prevention of uterine perforation during hysteroscopic treatment of severe Asherman's syndrome (Fig. 10.6).

10.3 Preoperative USG Assessment of Myometrial Thickness: To Guide the Amount of Adhesiolysis

Preoperative Ultrasound-Guided (USG) measurement of the myometrial thickness along the fundal, anterior, and posterior walls can guide the degree and direction of hysteroscopic adhesiolysis, obviating the need for concomitant laparoscopy. Sharma et al. [8] introduced "RR method" (named after main authors' names); this refers to the measurement of myometrial thicknesses at the fundal, anterior, and posterior walls that guides the amount and direction of hysteroscopic adhesiolysis and lateral metroplasty. They analyzed 21 women with Asherman's syndrome; all underwent preoperative USG measurement of the myometrial thickness; none required laparoscopic assistance during hysteroscopic adhesiolysis; and no perforation or false passage occurred.

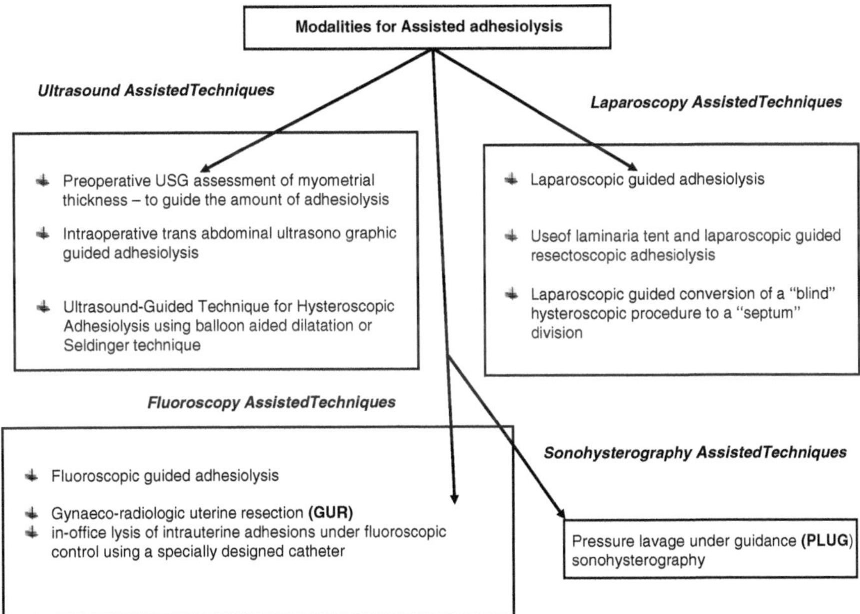

Fig. 10.6 Modalities for assisted adhesiolysis

10.4 Intraoperative Transabdominal Ultrasonographic Guided Adhesiolysis

Transabdominal ultrasound guidance has been increasingly used to replace laparoscopic guidance during hysteroscopic division of intrauterine adhesions, especially in women with severe intrauterine adhesions. When there are severe adhesions in the uterine cavity, it may be very difficult to identify the cavity without ultrasound.

Transabdominal ultrasonography provides efficient monitoring of the hysteroscopic procedure and guides the telescope towards the uterine cavity, even when the adhesions may have completely or almost completely obliterated the uterine cavity.

10.4.1 Advantages

1. The availability of ultrasound scan and its noninvasive nature; however, uterine perforation has been reported in as many as 5% of cases.
2. Can aid hysteroscopically directed division of severe IUAs and enable concurrent inspection of the pelvic organs.
3. Reduces iatrogenic perforation and false passages.

10.5 Laparoscopic Guided Adhesiolysis

Laparoscopic guided hysteroscopic adhesiolysis is commonly performed, particularly if the adhesions are dense. Lateral perforation of the uterus may cause significant bleeding, compared with central perforations. When the uterine wall becomes unduly thin, it will permit transmission of light across the uterine wall, and there will be a bulge over the remaining serosal layer, which signifies that further hysteroscopic surgery must immediately stop. However, with laparoscopic guidance, it is often too late to prevent the perforation. Nevertheless, it has the advantage of detecting the perforation immediately, preventing any further trauma to pelvic organs. Laparoscopy may also provide an opportunity to inspect the pelvis and to diagnose and treat any concurrent pathology such as endometriosis or adhesions and might reduce damage to the intestines as these are seen and moved out of the way.

10.6 Laparoscopic Guided Conversion of a "Blind" Hysteroscopic Procedure to a "Septum" Division

Conversion of a "blind" hysteroscopic procedure to a "septum" division: McComb and Wagner [9] used a variant hysteroscopic technique in six patients with severe intrauterine adhesions. The indication in all the cases was lack of communication between the cornua and the cervical canal as shown by hysterosalpingography (HSG). This method was performed hysteroscopically with concomitant laparoscopic guidance. A 5 mm hysteroscope was introduced with fluid used as the distending medium. A Pratt cervical dilator (gauge 13F) was passed through the cervix with the curved tip pointing laterally towards the uterine cornu. The dilator was aligned with the plane of the uterine corpus. The limit of passage was determined by the bulging of the cornua as seen by laparoscopy. This maneuver was performed bilaterally for a completely obliterated cavity. Thus, bilateral passage of the cervical dilator converted the obliterated uterine cavity into the configuration of a uterine "septum." The scar was cut with hysteroscopic scissors in side-to-side swaths, from one lateral passage to the other, until the fundus was reached and the uterine cavity had been liberated. In all six patients, regular menstruation was restored. Five women achieved conception, of whom four had live births. Three perforations and one hemorrhage were encountered among the six women. All the perforations were central. Postoperative HSG showed that the uterine cavity was normal.

10.7 Use of Laminaria Tent and Laparoscopic Guided Resectoscopic Adhesiolysis

Chen et al. [7] described the use of a laminaria tent followed by laparoscopic guided hysteroscopic adhesiolysis in seven patients. The laminaria tents consisted of a 6 cm length of dried kelp stalk, approximately 2 mm in diameter, with a string attached through a hole drilled 6 mm from the larger end. It was used to distend the short, narrow, scarred cervical cavity, thus facilitating the insertion of the transcervical resectoscope. Initially one or two of the tents were inserted into the cervix and left in situ with a vaginal pack for 24 hours. At the end of this time, the tents were replaced with 3–4 new tents, which were now placed within the uterine cavity itself and were removed 24 hours later. Gentle and gradual dilation of the cervical canal ensued as the laminaria absorbed fluid and gradually swelled after insertion. Hysteroscopic lysis of intrauterine adhesions was then performed under general anesthesia with a continuous-flow resectoscope. Simultaneous laparoscopy was used to guide the surgery. No intraoperative complications were recorded among the small number of women who participated in the study ($n = 7$). All their patients achieved normal menstruation after treatment, and a normal uterine cavity was demonstrated on repeat HSG.

They concluded that the management of severe uterine synechiae with a laminaria tent and transcervical laparoscopic guided resectoscope is a safe and appropriate treatment for severe adhesions.

10.8 Fluoroscopy-Guided Adhesiolysis

10.8.1 Advantages

1. It helps to delineate free areas above or behind the adhesions and reduce the incidence of a false passageway, and can be performed simultaneously with hysteroscopy.

2. It includes use of a narrow hysteroscope, reduced risk of uterine perforation, and reduced risk of visceral damage should perforation occur, because no energy source is applied.

10.8.2 Disadvantages

1. This technique exposes the patient to ionizing radiation.
2. It is costly and technically challenging.

Broome JD et al. [10] performed fluoroscopically guided hysteroscopic division of adhesions in severe Asherman's syndrome. Since 1984, approximately 55 women with severe Asherman's syndrome had undergone this procedure. All patients required at least two procedures, and one woman required six. There have been two cases of uneventful perforation with the Tuohy needle, and all women resumed menstruation. No serious complications have occurred.

Severe Asherman's syndrome refers to stage III disease according to the American Fertility Society, with obliteration of the uterine cavity and inability to visualize isolated pockets of the intrauterine cavity, which makes safe and effective hysteroscopic division of adhesions difficult, if not impossible.

Thomson AJ et al. [11] included 30 patients with Asherman's syndrome (13% AFS grade I, 43% AFS grade II, and 43% AFS grade III) for fluoroscopic assisted adhesiolysis. Prior to treatment, 60% of patients were amenorrheic. The median number of procedures per patient was 1.5 (range 1–6), and the mean length of the procedure was 42 min (range 10–70 min). After treatment, 96% had regular menses. Seventeen patients attempted to conceive after surgery, and 9 (53%) were successful. They concluded that hysteroscopic synechiolysis under image intensifier control appears to be an effective treatment for Asherman's syndrome.

10.8.3 Technique

A 16-gauge, 80 mm Tuohy needle is introduced into the endocervical canal alongside a 5 mm diagnostic hysteroscope. The surgeon probes the area beyond the adhesion with the needle. Ultravist 76.9% is injected through the needle under fluoroscopic and hysteroscopic control. Hidden pockets of endometrium can be located radiographically, a passageway is created using the needle, and subsequent division of adhesions is performed under direct vision with hysteroscopic scissors.

10.9 Gynecoradiologic Uterine Resection (GUR)

Seth Levrant et al. [12] described in-office lysis of intrauterine adhesions under fluoroscopic control using a specially designed catheter. The initial hysterosalpingography was performed with a commercially available uterine catheter that seals off the uterine cavity before injection of contrast. If intrauterine adhesions were diagnosed, an immediate attempt at lysis was made using the catheter's balloon-tip or hysteroscopic scissors, which were inserted through the main port of the catheter. The procedures were carried out using a paracervical block or intravenous analgesia.

Seventeen patients underwent lysis of intrauterine adhesions. In 13 patients (9 mild, 3 moderate, and 1 severe), the adhesions were lysed successfully (81.2%). Among those, nine procedures were performed with the balloon and four with scissors. In four cases (two moderate and two severe), lysis of adhesions was only partially successful. These procedures had to be abandoned prematurely because of patient discomfort before attempting the use of scissors ($n = 1$), extravasation of dye into the myometrium making visualization difficult ($n = 1$), and thick, fibrotic adhesions that were resistant to scissors ($n = 2$).

They concluded that in-office lysis of intrauterine adhesions under gynecoradiologic control could be carried out safely in the majority of patients, using minimally invasive techniques. The potential cost savings in comparison with endoscopic procedures, which require utilization of expensive operating room time, are especially relevant in today's cost-conscious managed care environment. Only failures of in-office procedures would reach the operating room under the algorithm proposed here.

10.10 Pressure Lavage Under Guidance (PLUG)

Coccia et al. [13] described a technique based on sonohysterography in which a continuous intrauterine injection of saline solution led to mechanical disruption of intrauterine adhesions. They included five patients with mild adhesions and obtained satisfactory lysis of the adhesions and restoration of menses. However, two patients with moderate adhesions underwent repeated treatment by hysteroscopy several months after the procedure because of the reformation of filmy adhesions. One out of the seven patients achieved pregnancy. They concluded that this technique is suitable for mild adhesions.

10.11 Ultrasound-Guided Technique for Hysteroscopic Adhesiolysis Using Balloon-Aided Dilatation or Seldinger Technique

Kriseman M et al. [14] described a novel approach of using ultrasound (US)-guided balloon dilation to safely and effectively treat intrauterine adhesions and to decrease the risk of perforation. They reported three patients, one with cervical stenosis and two with Asherman's syndrome, who underwent US-guided adhesiolysis. Access to the uterine cavity was obtained by either direct balloon-aided dilation or US-guided Seldinger technique, followed by balloon-aided dilation to enter the endometrial cavity and disrupt intrauterine/intracervical adhesions.

The treatment of Asherman's syndrome still poses a challenge. Since the condition most often follows the curettage of a pregnant or recently pregnant uterus, this should be avoided where possible, with recourse to medical termination of pregnancy where feasible. If surgical evacuation is inevitable, the surgeon should be as gentle as possible. Hysteroscopy still remains the gold standard in the diagnosis and treatment of Asherman's syndrome. More research is needed regarding the optimum adhesion prevention strategy.

10.12 Prevention of Adhesion Reformation

Adhesion reformation is common following hysteroscopic adhesiolysis. Hanstede et al. [15] found a recurrence in 174 out of 638 patients (27.3%) who had hysteroscopic adhesiolysis. As expected, the recurrence rate was much higher in patients with more severe disease.

It is vital that steps are taken aimed at preventing the recurrence of IUA. There are various strategies but no single one has been proven to be effective.

10.13 AAGL and ESGE Practice Guidelines, 2017 [16]

Adjunctive interventions to aid adhesiolysis include ultrasound, fluoroscopy, and laparoscopy. There are no data to suggest that these prevent perforation or improve surgical outcomes and are likely dependent on clinical skills and availability. However, when such an approach is used in appropriately selected patients, it may minimize the consequences if perforation occurs: **Level B**.

Key Points

1. Hysteroscopic division of intrauterine adhesions may be technically difficult, especially if the adhesions are dense.
2. The efficiency and safety of hysteroscopic surgery for severe Asherman's syndrome may be improved if the procedure is done under guidance or assistance.
3. Modalities for assisted adhesiolysis are ultrasonography, laparoscopy, fluoroscopy, and sonohysterography.
4. Mild-to-moderate cases might be managed on an outpatient basis without any need for anesthesia, while severe cases are generally managed under general or regional anesthesia.
5. Cautery is more likely to cause damage to the endometrium compared with scissors but is associated with better ability to secure hemostasis.

References

1. Tao Z, Duan H. Expression of adhesion-related cytokines in the uterine fluid after transcervical resection of adhesion. Zhonghua Fu Chan KeZaZhi. 2012;47:734–7.
2. Schenker JG, Margalioth EJ. Intrauterine adhesions: an updated appraisal. Fertil Steril. 1982;37(5):593–610.
3. Al-Inany H. Intrauterine adhesions: an update. Acta Obstet Gynecol Scand. 2001;80:986–93.

4. Sugimoto O. Diagnostic and therapeutic hysteroscopy for traumatic intrauterine adhesions. Am J Obstet Gynecol. 1978;131:539–47.
5. Okohue JE, Onuh SO, Akaba GO, Shaibu I, Wada I, Ikimalo JI. A 3 years review of hysteroscopy in a private hospital in Nigeria. World J Laparosc Surg. 2009;2:26–9.
6. Dreisler E, Kjer JJ. Asherman's syndrome: current perspectives on diagnosis and management. Int J Women's Health. 2019;1:191–8.
7. Chen FP, Soong YK, Hui YL. Successful treatment of severe uterine synechiae with transcervical resectoscopy combined with laminaria tent. Hum Reprod. 1997;12:943–7. https://doi.org/10.1093/humrep/12.5.943.
8. Sharma R, Manchanda R, Chandil N. Revisiting diagnostic and therapeutic challenges in Asherman's syndrome: a retrospective analysis of 5 years. Int J Curr Res. 2018;10(8):72429–34.
9. McComb PF, Wagner BL. Simplified therapy for Asherman's syndrome. Fertil Steril. 1997;68:1047–50.
10. Broome JD, Vancaillie TG. Fluoroscopically guided hysteroscopic division of adhesions in severe Asherman syndrome. Obstet Gynecol. 1999;93(6):1041–3.
11. Thomson AJ, Abbott JA, Kingston A, Lenart M, Vancaillie TG. Fluoroscopically guided synechiolysis for patients with Asherman's syndrome: menstrual and fertility outcomes. Fertil Steril. 2007;87(2):405–10.
12. Levrant S, Hoxsey R, Rinehart J, Gleicher N. Lysis of intrauterine adhesions using gynecoradiologic techniques. Fertil Steril. 1997;68(4):658–62.
13. Coccia ME, Becattini C, Bracco GL, Pampaloni F, Bargelli G, Scarselli G. Pressure lavage under ultrasound guidance: a new approach for outpatient treatment of intrauterine adhesions. Fertil Steril. 2001;75:601–6.
14. Kriseman M, Schutt A, Appleton J, Pillai A, George V, Zarutskie PW. A novel ultrasound-guided technique for hysteroscopic adhesiolysis in high-risk patients. J Ultrasound Med. 2019;38(5):1383–7. https://doi.org/10.1002/jum.14815.
15. Hanstede MMF, van der Meij E, Goedemans L, Emmanuel MH. Results of centralized Asherman surgery, 2003–2013. Fertil Steril. 2015;104(6):1561–8.
16. AAGL Elevating Gynecologic Surgery. AAGL practice report: practice guidelines on intrauterine adhesions developed in collaboration with the European Society of Gynaecological Endoscopy (ESGE). J Minim Invasive Gynecol. 2017;24(5):695–705.

Postoperative Care (Hormonal Therapy, Physical Barriers, Vasodilators, Antibiotics)

11

Sarah Gustapane, Bruno Francesco Barba, and Andrea Tinelli

Intrauterine adhesions (IUAs) can occur after mechanical or infectious injury to the endometrium. Normal endometrial repair occurs without scar formation; however, in some women, these normal repair mechanisms are aberrant, resulting in IUA formation. The exact alteration in repair mechanisms is not well understood; however, it likely involves hypoxia, reduced neovascularization, and altered expression of adhesion-associated cytokines.

IUAs can lead to partial or complete closure of the uterine cavity, which may result in symptoms including abnormal menstruation, infertility, and pelvic pain (Fig. 11.1a, b).

The IUAs have been studied and classified since the 1978 (*classification is described in detail in Chap. 4*).

Although numerous observational studies suggest potential benefit with the use of anti-adhesion therapies (intrauterine device or balloon, hormonal treatment, barrier gels, or human amniotic membrane grafting) for decreasing IUAs, currently,

S. Gustapane
Department of Obstetrics and Gynecology, "Veris delli Ponti" Hospital, Scorrano, Lecce, Italy

B. F. Barba
Department of Obstetrics and Gynecology, Casa di Cura Salus s.r.l., Brindisi, Italy

A. Tinelli (✉)
Department of Obstetrics and Gynecology, "Veris delli Ponti" Hospital, Scorrano, Lecce, Italy

Division of Experimental Endoscopic Surgery, Imaging, Technology and Minimally Invasive Therapy, Vito Fazzi Hospital, Lecce, Italy

Laboratory of Human Physiology, Phystech BioMed School, Faculty of Biological and Medical Physics, Moscow Institute of Physics and Technology (State University), Dolgoprudny, Moscow, Russia

R. Manchanda (ed.), *Intra Uterine Adhesions*,
https://doi.org/10.1007/978-981-33-4145-6_11

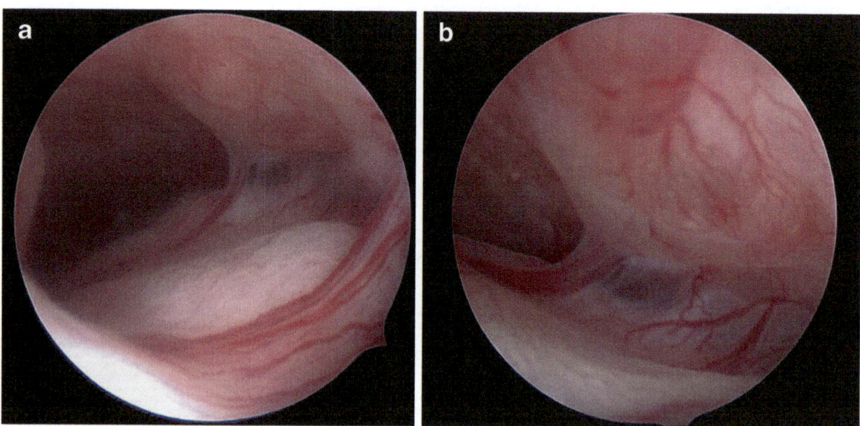

Fig. 11.1 (**a**, **b**) Mild intrauterine adhesions

there are no strong recommendations in favor of the use of anti-adhesion therapies after operative hysteroscopy.

At present the effectiveness of the anti-adhesion treatment following operative hysteroscopy for decreasing IUAs remains uncertain as suggested by the Cochrane Review of 2017 [1] because of the low quality of the evidence [1].

The pathogenesis of IUAs is related to many physiopathologic mechanisms, such as the lesion of the basal layer of the endometrium, caused by curettage, hysteroscopic surgery, uterine artery embolization, B-lynch sutures, abdominal myomectomy, hysteroscopic myomectomy, genital tuberculosis, and surgical treatment of Mullerian anomalies. They could cause the partial or complete obstruction of the cervix and the uterine cavity, with the consequent obstruction of sperm transport into the cervix, impaired embryo migration within the uterine cavity, and failure of embryo implantation [2, 3].

The occurrence of new adhesions after primary hysteroscopic adhesiolysis is so much frequent and the recurrence rate is associated with the grade of adherences (Figs. 11.2 and 11.3).

According the classification system of the former European Society of Hysteroscopy, Hanstede et al. found 21–25% recurrence with grade 1–2 adherences, 29.1% with grade 3, 38.5% with grade 4, and 41.9% with grade 5 [4].

There are several methods for secondary prevention, such as the use of estrogen, intrauterine device, Foley catheter, antibiotics, hyaluronic acid, and stem cell treatment used alone or in combination with each other.

The Cochrane Review (2017) of Bosteels et al. compared a device versus no treatment (two studies; 90 women), hormonal treatment versus no treatment or placebo (two studies; 136 women), device combined with hormonal treatment versus no treatment (one study; 20 women), barrier gel versus no treatment (five studies; 464 women), device with graft versus device without graft (three studies; 190

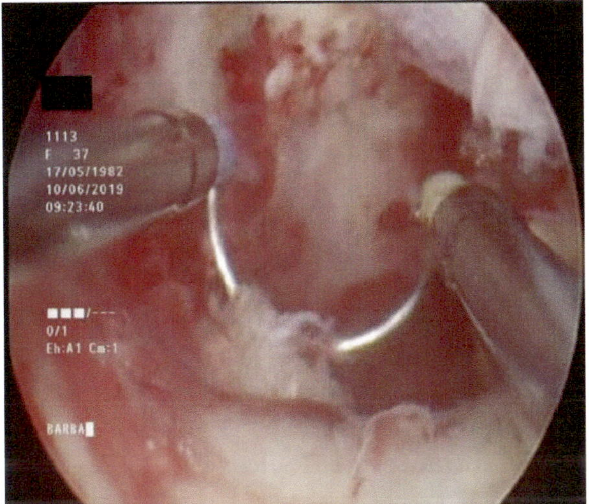

Fig. 11.2 Resectoscopic adhesiolysis

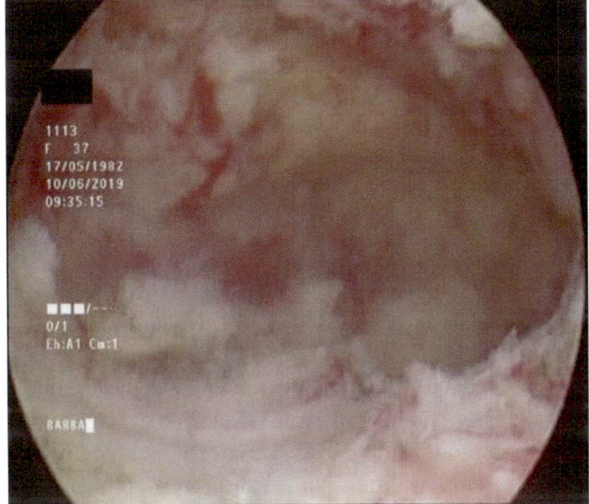

Fig. 11.3 Shows adhesion formation following primary hysteroscopic adhesiolysis

women), one type of device versus another device (one study; 201 women), gel combined with hormonal treatment and antibiotics versus hormonal treatment with antibiotics (one study; 52 women), and device combined with gel versus device (one study; 120 women) [1].

They concluded that the quality of the evidence ranged from very low to low. The effectiveness of anti-adhesion treatment for improving key reproductive outcomes or for decreasing IUAs following operative hysteroscopy in subfertile women remains uncertain.

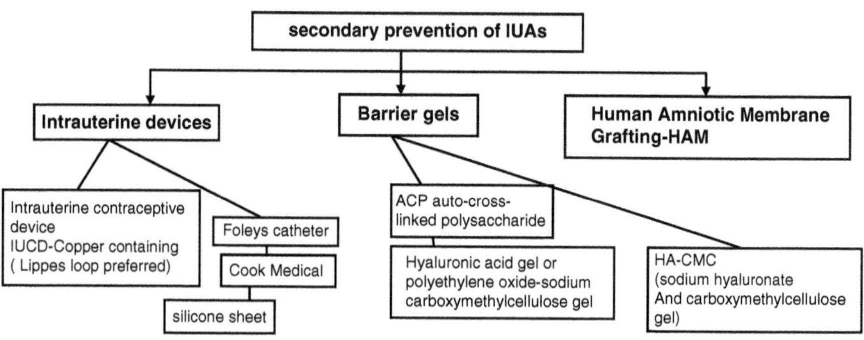

Fig. 11.4 Secondary prevention of IUAs

11.1 Intrauterine Devices (Fig. 11.5a–f)

The characteristics of an intrauterine device (IUD) to prevent intrauterine adhesion formation should be the tolerability of the device, the suppression of IUA formation, and the restoring of healing of the endometrium. There are several observational studies that recommended the insertion of a device after lysis of IUAs such as IUD and Foley catheter balloon after lysis of IUAs or septoplasty. The IUD may provide a physical barrier between the uterine walls, separating the endometrial layers [5]. There are different kinds of IUD with particular characteristics and mechanism of actions: copper-containing IUD provokes an excessive inflammatory reaction, and T-shaped IUD may have a surface too small to maintain separation of the uterine walls; instead the loop IUD is generally considered the IUD of choice for treatment of IUAs; however, it is not available in many geographic areas [6]. The Cook Medical balloon (Indianapolis, IN, USA) has been designed to be a heart-shaped intrauterine balloon for prevention of secondary intrauterine adhesions thanks to its triangular shape, which conforms to the configuration of a normal uterus and maintains separation at the margins of uterine cavity [7].

In a randomized controlled trial, Lin et al. compared the efficacy of intrauterine balloon (removed after 7 days) and IUD demonstrating similar efficacy [8].

The use of other mechanical barriers is also suggested for the prevention of secondary adhesions. Orhue et al. compared an IUD with a pediatric Foley catheter and found that the catheter was a safer and more effective adjunctive method of treatment of IUA compared with the IUD. The persistent posttreatment amenorrhea and hypomenorrhea occurred less frequently in the Foley catheter group (18.6%) than in the IUD group (37.3%) ($P < 0.03$), and the conception rate in the catheter group was 33.9% compared with 22.5% in the IUD group. The need for repeated treatment was also significantly less in the Foley catheter group [9].

Recently, Shi et al. compared the efficacy of intermittent intrauterine balloon dilatation versus standard care in the prevention of adhesion reformation in 200 patients with moderate-to-severe IUAs who underwent hysteroscopic adhesiolysis. In this randomized controlled trial, the balloon group received intrauterine balloon

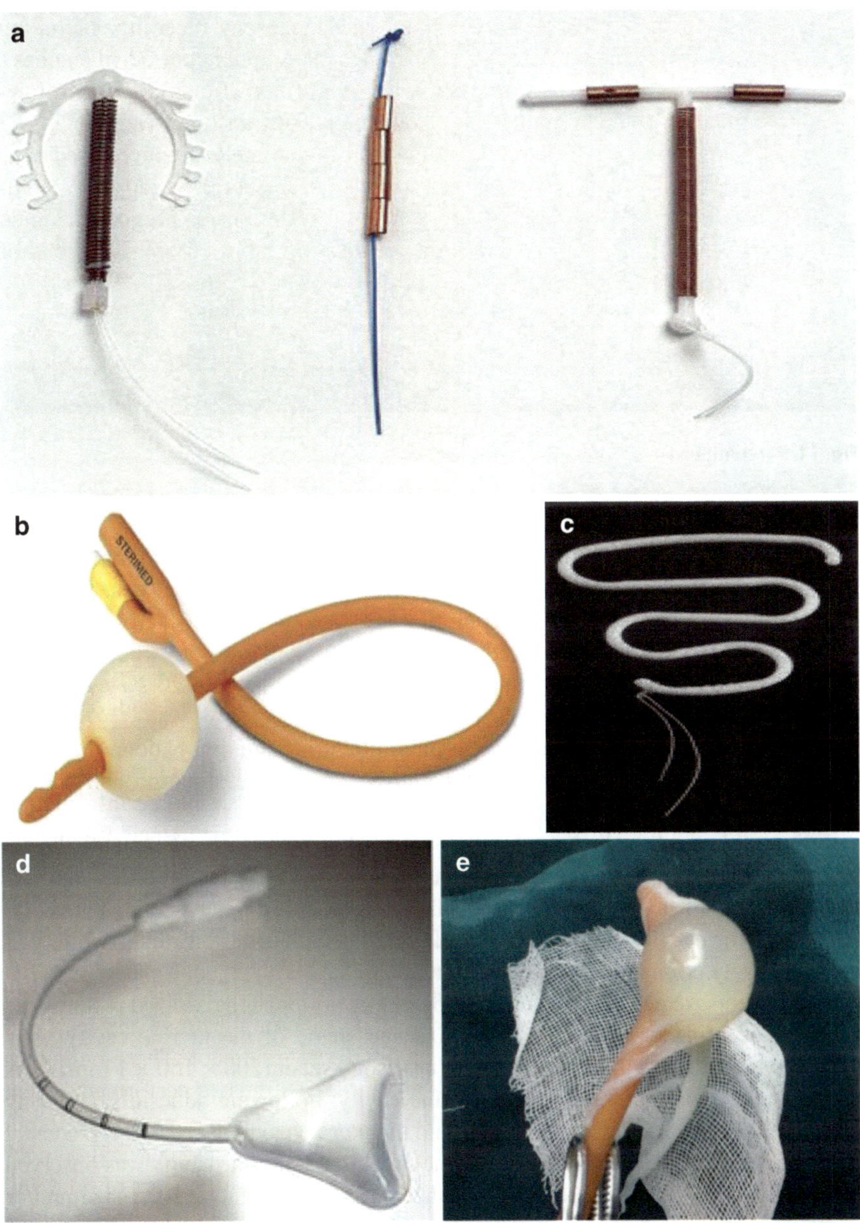

Fig. 11.5 (**a**) Copper T. (**b**) Foley catheter. (**c**) Lippes loop. (**d**) Cook Medical balloon. (**e**) Foley catheter with mounted amnion. (**f**) Silicon sheet cut into shape of uterus

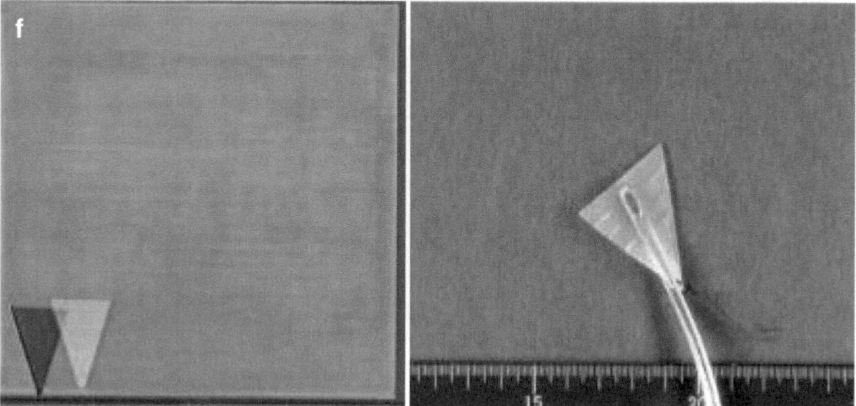

Fig. 11.5 (continued)

dilatation therapy at 2 and 6 weeks after surgery, whereas the control group did not. A total of 191 patients successfully completed the study protocol (94 cases for the balloon group and 97 cases for the control group). According to hysteroscopic evaluation at the 8th week, the overall adhesion reformation rate was significantly lower in patients in the balloon group than patients in the control group (20.2% vs. 40.2%, respectively; $P < 0.05$).

This study shows that postoperative intermittent intrauterine balloon dilatation therapy can significantly reduce postoperative adhesion reformation and significantly increase menstruation flow [10].

Silicone sheet: Atsushi Azumaguchi et al. [11] evaluated the efficacy of silicone sheet as a new type of barrier for preventing adhesion reformation following hysteroscopic adhesiolysis of intrauterine adhesions (IUAs). Hysteroscopic adhesiolysis was performed for 36 patients with IUAs. The adhesion reformation rate was retrospectively compared between 26 patients treated with silicone sheet (group 1) and 10 patients treated with an intrauterine device wrapped in oxidized regenerated cellulose as a barrier (group 2). The size and shape of the uterine cavity were observed by hysterosalpingography, and a silicone sheet ($200 \times 150 \times 1$ mm^3) was cut to fit the size and shape of the uterine cavity. Following adhesiolysis during surgery, the silicone sheet was inserted into the uterine cavity using small placental forceps, and then the fitness of the silicone sheet in the uterine cavity was observed by hysteroscopy. When necessary, the sheet was pulled out, and the size and/or shape corrected as many times as needed. After confirming an appropriate fit, six slits were made in the sheet to prevent the sheet from slipping out of the uterine cavity, nylon thread was threaded through a small hole in the lower part of the sheet to allow easy retraction after insertion, and the device was placed in the uterine cavity (Fig. 11.5f). The adhesion reformation rate was significantly lower in group 1 (4/26, 15.4%) than in group 2 (4/10, 40.0%; $P = 0.03$), although the pregnancy rate (14/20, 70.0% vs. 5/10, 50.0%; $P = 0.28$) and miscarriage rate (2/14, 14.3% vs. 1/5,

20.0%; $P = 0.72$) were not significantly different. They concluded that the use of silicone sheets appears to be effective for preventing adhesion reformation following hysteroscopic adhesiolysis of IUAs.

11.1.1 Barrier Gels

Several adhesion barriers are reported to be useful in reducing the risk of adhesion recurrence after surgical treatment of IUAs [12–14]. Use of biodegradable gel surgical barriers is based on the principle of keeping adjacent wound surfaces mechanically separate [15]. The exact mechanisms by which ACP (auto-cross-linked polysaccharide) and HA-CMC (sodium hyaluronate and carboxymethylcellulose gel) can reduce adhesion reformation are not well known but may be related to "hydro-flotation" or "siliconizing" effects. Hyaluronic acid gel or polyethylene oxide-sodium carboxymethylcellulose gel for the prevention of intrauterine adherences has been investigated demonstrating conflicting results. Acunzo et al. found a significant effect of hyaluronic acid compared to no treatment (14% vs. 32%) [14]. Instead Lin et al. demonstrated that the balloon and IUCD were more effective than hyaluronic acid [8].

Ducarne et al. compared application of ACP gel (30 women) versus no gel (24 women) at the end of an operative hysteroscopic procedure performed to treat myomas, polyps, uterine septa, or IUAs, finding no statistically significant differences between comparison groups in the rate of adhesion formation or in mean adhesion scores and severity of adhesions [16].

11.1.2 Human Amniotic Membrane Grafting

Human amniotic membrane (HAM) is a rich source of biologically active factors, supports epithelialization, and exhibits anti-fibrotic, anti-inflammatory, antiangiogenic, and antimicrobial features, as the ophthalmology studies suggest [17]. The clinical use of HAM in regenerative medicine is currently increasing. In the field of obstetrics and gynecology its use is limited for vaginoplasty and radical vulvectomy and for prevention of postoperative intra-abdominal adhesion. HAM acts as a biologically active mechanical barrier to suppress adhesion formation while promoting endometrial healing [18], through regeneration of epithelium facilitating migration of epithelial cells, reinforcing adhesion of the basal epithelium, promoting epithelial cell differentiation [19], preventing cellular apoptosis [20], producing factors, or creating a microenvironment for effective tissue repair and endometrial regeneration, possibly by stimulating endogenous stem cells [21].

According to a randomized controlled trial of Zheng et al. including 300 patients, which evaluated the ability of HAM to prevent the recurrence of IUAs after hysteroscopic adhesiolysis, the use of HAM increased menstrual blood volume (mean difference 6.15, 95% CI 4.20–8.11; $P < 0.001$) but failed to improve the rate of intrauterine adhesion recurrence or spontaneous abortion [22].

Yan et al. in a network meta-analysis of randomized controlled trials have found a significant advantage with the use of freeze-dried amniotic agents plus a balloon to reduce IUA recurrence and IUA scores after adhesiolysis [23].

A prospective randomized controlled trial conducted among 88 women with severe IUA who underwent hysteroscopic adhesiolysis analyzed the efficacy of freeze-dried amnion graft that covered the balloon portion of the Foley catheter for prevention of IUAs. Also, this study concluded that the use of HAM was effective in improving menstruation, but the rates of IUA reformation and pregnancy were not significantly different [24].

11.1.3 Vasodilators

Vasodilators have been proposed to increase endometrial receptivity and endometrial thickness in order to enhance the chances for successful assisted pregnancy. But evidence was insufficient to show whether vasodilators increase the live birth rate [25].

Many studies described the use of medications to increase vascular flow to endometrium such as aspirin, nitroglycerine, and sildenafil citrate in order to increase vascular perfusion to the endometrium and enable pregnancy. Zinger reported two cases of woman with a history of a postpartum uterine curettage, with inadequate endometrium thickness after surgical resection of IUAs that are treated with sildenafil citrate, and with the results of having achieved pregnancy [26].

However, the number of women treated using these therapies remains small, and because all such treatments are off label, these medications cannot be endorsed outside of rigorous research protocols.

11.1.4 Antibiotics

Transcervical intrauterine procedures entail a risk of contamination by vaginal flora and might result in infection. However, there is no clear recommendation in the literature on whether it is necessary to use prophylactic antibiotics for minor operative procedures such as dilatation and curettage for evacuation of conceptive products, fractional curettage for abnormal uterine bleeding, hysterosalpingography for infertility evaluation, and hysteroscopy for intrauterine cavity diagnosis and treatment.

The Cochrane of 2013 regarding the prophylactic antibiotics for transcervical intrauterine procedures versus placebo concluded that there are no randomized controlled trials that assess the effects of prophylactic antibiotics on infection complications and therefore it is not possible to draw any conclusions [27]. However, when obvious infection is seen, antibiotics are mandatory.

In India genital tuberculosis appears to be an important and common cause of IUA causing primary and secondary infertility with various grades of adhesions [28] and so it is important to investigate the patients who come from those areas.

11.1.5 Hormonal Therapy

Already in 1964 Wood and Pena hypothesized the beneficial effects of estrogen therapy on endometrial regeneration after surgical treatment for IUAs [29]. Postoperative treatment with estrogen in order to promote the regeneration of the endometrium has been recommended in several studies, either as estrogen only [30, 31] or with IUD [8, 32–38] or Foley catheter [31, 32, 38].

In several studies different regimens consisting of estrogen with or without a progestogen have been used [6]. There are no comparative studies that examine dosage, administration, or combinations of hormones [2]. In a recent randomized study, 4 and 10 mg estradiol orally was compared. No superior effect of the high dosage was demonstrated [39]. When comparing 2 and 6 mg in a prospective randomized trial, no benefit was demonstrated in the 6 mg arm.

In the randomized controlled trials of Farhi et al., 60 women undergoing dilatation and curettage during the first trimester of pregnancy were allocated to receive estrogen combined with progestogen or no treatment [40]. The authors have found that women in the intervention group had a significantly thicker endometrium compared with women in the control group (8.4 with intervention vs. 6.7 mm with no treatment; $P = 0.02$) and so they concluded that postoperative hormonal treatment may be useful for IUA prevention following curettage. Nevertheless, this study does not report the data about pregnancy rates and IUA recurrence [40]. The systematic review of Johary et al. concluded that estrogen therapy may be beneficial for women with IUAs, but as adjunctive therapy combined with other anti-adhesion strategies [41]. Also, in three prospective randomized studies, the administration of oral estrogen did not reduce the risk of IUAs [35, 42, 43].

Sravani Chithra et al. [44] (2016) conducted a retrospective analysis of 101 women with IUAs. They proposed and recommended the doses of conjugated estrogen and progesterone according to severity of AS, showing good results (Table 11.1).

11.2 Guidelines for Secondary Prevention of Intrauterine Adhesions: AAGL/ESGE 2017 [45]

1. The use of an IUD, stent, or catheter appears to reduce the rate of postoperative adhesion reformation. There are limited data regarding subsequent fertility outcomes when these barriers are used: **Grade A**.
2. The risk of infection appears to be minimal when a solid barrier is used compared with no treatment: **Grade A**.

Table 11.1 Dosage of conjugated estrogen and progesterone according to severity of AS

Severity	Conjugated estrogen (21 days)	Medroxyprogesterone acetate (7 days)
Mild	0.625 mg twice a day	10 mg twice a day
Moderate	1.25 mg twice a day	10 mg twice a day
Severe	1.25 mg four times a day	10 mg twice a day

3. There is no evidence to support or refute the use of preoperative, intraoperative, or postoperative antibiotic therapy in surgical treatment of IUAs: **Grade C**.
4. If an IUD is used postoperatively, it should be inert and have a large surface area such as a Lippes loop. Intrauterine devices that contain progestin or copper should not be used after surgical division of IUAs: **Grade C.**
5. Semisolid barriers such as hyaluronic acid and auto-cross-linked hyaluronic acid gel reduce adhesion reformation. At this time, their effect on posttreatment pregnancy rates is unknown: **Grade A**.
6. Following hysteroscopic directed adhesiolysis, postoperative hormone treatment using estrogen, with or without progestin, may reduce the recurrence of IUAs: **Grade B**.
7. The role of medications designed as adjuvants to improve vascular flow to the endometrium has not been established. Consequently, they should not be used outside of rigorous research protocols: **Grade C**.
8. Stem cell treatment may ultimately provide an effective adjuvant approach to the treatment of Asherman syndrome; however, evidence is very limited and this treatment should not be offered outside of rigorous research protocols: **Grade C**.

Key Points

1. Many devices, used alone or in combination, have been proposed to prevent IUA formation after intrauterine procedures.
2. At present it is difficult to establish which approach is the best, due to the heterogeneity of the studies, the contrasting results reported, and the different outcomes investigated.
3. To avoid adhesion relapse, it would seem to be recommendable the use of balloon catheters and IUD with adjunctive estrogen therapy.
4. More research is needed to assess the best approach to prevent adhesions in order to increase reproductive chances and if pregnancy occurs to reduce obstetrics risk such as miscarriage, preterm birth, abnormal placentation, and intrauterine growth restriction.

References

1. Bosteels J, Weyers S, D'Hooghe TM, Torrance H, Broekmans FJ, Chua SJ, Mol BWJ. Anti-adhesion therapy following operative hysteroscopy for treatment of female subfertility. Cochrane Database Syst Rev. 2017;11(11):CD011110.
2. Deans R, Abbott J. Review of intrauterine adhesions. J Minim Invasive Gynecol. 2010;17:555–69.
3. Dreisler E, Kjer JJ. Asherman's syndrome: current perspectives on diagnosis and management. Int J Women's Health. 2019;11:191–8.
4. Hanstede MMF, van der Meij E, Goedemans L, Emanuel MH. Results of centralized Asherman surgery, 2003–2013. Fertil Steril. 2015;104(6):15611568.
5. Xu W, Zhang Y, Yang Y, Zhang S, Lin X. Effect of early second-look hysteroscopy on reproductive outcomes after hysteroscopic adhesiolysis in patients with intrauterine adhesion, a retrospective study in China. Int J Surg. 2018;50:49–54.

6. Kodaman PH, Arici A. Intra-uterine adhesions and fertility outcome: how to optimize success? Curr Opin Obstet Gynecol. 2007;19(3):207–14.
7. March CM. Management of Asherman's syndrome. Reprod BioMed Online. 2011;23(1):63–76.
8. Orhue AAE, Aziken ME, Igbefoh JO. A comparison of two adjunctive treatments for intrauterine adhesions following lysis. Int J Gynaecol Obstet. 2003;82:49–56.
9. Lin XN, Zhou F, Wei ML, et al. Randomized, controlled trial comparing the efficacy of intrauterine balloon and intrauterine contraceptive device in the prevention of adhesion reformation after hysteroscopic adhesiolysis. Fertil Steril. 2015;104(1):235–40.
10. Shi X, Saravelos SH, Zhou Q, Huang X, Xia E, Li TC. Prevention of postoperative adhesion reformation by intermittent intrauterine balloon therapy: a randomised controlled trial. BJOG. 2019;126(10):1259–66.
11. Azumaguchi A, Henmi H, Saito T. Efficacy of silicone sheet as a personalized barrier for preventing adhesion reformation after hysteroscopic adhesiolysis of intrauterine adhesions. Reprod Med Biol. 2019;18:378–83.
12. Guida M, Acunzo G, Di Spiezio SA, et al. Effectiveness of auto-crosslinked hyaluronic acid gel in the prevention of intrauterine adhesions after hysteroscopic surgery: a prospective, randomized, controlled study. Hum Reprod. 2004;19:1461–4.
13. Tsapanos VS, Stathopoulou LP, Papathanassopoulou VS, Tzingounis VA. The role of Seprafilm bioresorbable membrane in the prevention and therapy of endometrial synechiae. J Biomed Mater Res. 2002;63:10–4.
14. Acunzo G, Guida M, Pellicano M, et al. Effectiveness of auto-cross-linked hyaluronic acid gel in the prevention of intrauterine adhesions after hysteroscopic adhesiolysis: a prospective, randomized, controlled study. Hum Reprod. 2003;18:1918–21.
15. Renier D, Bellato PA, Bellini D, Pavesio A, Pressato D, Borrione A. Pharmacokinetic behaviour of ACP gel, an autocrosslinked hyaluronan derivative, after intraperitoneal administration. Biomaterials. 2005;26:5368–74.
16. Ducarme G, Davitian C, Zarrouk S, Uzan M, Poncelet C. Interest of auto-crosslinked hyaluronic acid gel in the prevention of intrauterine adhesions after hysteroscopic surgery: a case-control study. J Gynecol Obstet Biol Reprod. 2006;35(7):691–5.
17. Jirsova K, Jones GLA. Amniotic membrane in ophthalmology: properties, preparation, storage and indications for grafting-a review. Cell Tissue Bank. 2017;18(2):193–204.
18. Amer MI, Abd-El-Maeboud KH. Amnion graft following hysteroscopic lysis of intrauterine adhesions. J Obstet Gynaecol Res. 2006;32(6):559–66.
19. Meller D, Tseng SC. Conjunctival epithelial cell differentiation on amniotic membrane. Invest Ophthalmol Vis Sci. 1999;40:878–86.
20. Hori J, Wang M, Kamiya K, Takahashi H, Sakuragawa N. Immunological characteristics of amniotic epithelium. Cornea. 2006;25(10 Suppl 1):S53–8.
21. Committee ACOG. on Practice Bulletins ACOG Practice Bulletin No. 74. Antibiotic prophylaxis for gynecologic procedures. Obstet Gynecol. 2006;108:225–34. https://doi.org/10.1097/00006250-200607000-00057.
22. Zheng F, Zhu B, Liu Y, Wang R, Cui Y. Meta-analysis of the use of amniotic membrane to prevent recurrence of intrauterine adhesion after hysteroscopic adhesiolysis. Int J Gynaecol Obstet. 2018;143(2):145–9.
23. Yan Y, Xu D. The effect of adjuvant treatment to prevent and treat intrauterine adhesions: a network meta-analysis of randomized controlled trials. J Minim Invasive Gynecol. 2018;25(4):589–99.
24. Gan L, Duan H, Sun FQ, Xu Q, Tang YQ, Wang S. Efficacy of freeze-dried amnion graft following hysteroscopic adhesiolysis of severe intrauterine adhesions. Int J Gynaecol Obstet. 2017;137(2):116–22.
25. Gutarra-Vilchez RB, Bonfill Cosp X, Glujovsky D, Viteri-García A, Runzer-Colmenares FM, Martinez-Zapata MJ. Vasodilators for women undergoing fertility treatment. Cochrane Database Syst Rev. 2018;10:CD010001.
26. Zinger M, Liu JH, Thomas MA. Successful use of vaginal sildenafil citrate in two infertility patients with Asherman's syndrome. J Women's Health. 2006;15:442–4.

27. Thinkhamrop J, Laopaiboon M, Lumbiganon P. Prophylactic antibiotics for transcervical intrauterine procedures. Cochrane Database Syst Rev. 2013;2013(5):CD005637.
28. Sharma JB, Roy KK, Pushparaj M, et al. Genital tuberculosis: an important cause of Asherman's syndrome in India. Arch Gynecol Obstet. 2008;277(1):37–41.
29. Wood J, Pena G. Treatment of traumatic uterine synechias. Int J Fertil. 1964;9:405–10.
30. Capella-Allouc S, Morsad F, Rongières-Bertrand C, Taylor S, Fernandez H. Hysteroscopic treatment of severe Asherman's syndrome and subsequent fertility. Hum Reprod. 1999;14(5):1230–3.
31. Dawood A, Al-Talib A, Tulandi T. Predisposing factors and treatment outcome of different stages of intrauterine adhesions. J Obstet Gynaecol Can. 2010;32(8):767–70.
32. March CM, Israel R, March AD. Hysteroscopic management of intrauterine adhesions. Am J Obstet Gynecol. 1978;130(6):653–7.
33. Chen L, Zhang H, Wang Q, et al. Reproductive outcomes in patients with intrauterine adhesions following hysteroscopic adhesiolysis: experience from the largest women's hospital in China. J Minim Invasive Gynecol. 2017;24(2):299–304.
34. Yu X, Yuhan L, Dongmei S, Enlan X, Tinchiu L. The incidence of postoperative adhesion following transection of uterine septum: a cohort study comparing three different adjuvant therapies. Eur J Obstet Gynecol Reprod Biol. 2016;201:61–4.
35. Roy KK, Negi N, Subbaiah M, Kumar S, Sharma JB, Singh N. Effectiveness of estrogen in the prevention of intrauterine adhesions after hysteroscopic septal resection: a prospective, randomized study. J Obstet Gynaecol Res. 2014;40(4):1085–8.
36. Zikopoulos KA, Kolibianakis EM, Platteau P, et al. Live delivery rates in subfertile women with Asherman's syndrome after hysteroscopic adhesiolysis using the resectoscope or the Versapoint system. Reprod BioMed Online. 2004;8(6):720–5.
37. Myers EM, Hurst BS. Comprehensive management of severe Asherman syndrome and amenorrhea. Fertil Steril. 2012;97(1):160–4.
38. Salma U, Xue M, Md Sayed AS, Xu D. Efficacy of intrauterine device in the treatment of intrauterine adhesions. Biomed Res Int. 2014;2014(5):1–15.
39. Liu L, Huang X, Xia E, Zhang X, Li TC, Liu Y. A cohort study comparing 4 mg and 10 mg daily doses of postoperative oestradiol therapy to prevent adhesion reformation after hysteroscopic adhesiolysis. Hum Fertil. 2018;48:1–7.
40. Farhi J, Bar-Hava I, Homburg R, Dicker D, Ben-Rafael Z. Induced regeneration of endometrium following curettage for abortion: a comparative study. Hum Reprod. 1993;8:1143.
41. Johary J, Xue M, Zhu X, Xu D, Palani VP. The efficacy of estrogen therapy in patients with intrauterine adhesions: a systematic review. J Minim Invasive Gynecol. 2014;21(1):44–54.
42. Tonguc EA, Var T, Yilmaz N, Batioglu S. Intrauterine device or estrogen treatment after hysteroscopic uterine septum resection. Int J Gynaecol Obstet. 2010;109(3):226–9.
43. Dabirashrafi H, Mohammad K, Moghadami-Tabrizi N, Zandinejad K, Moghadami-Tabrizi M. Is estrogen necessary after hysteroscopic incision of the uterine septum? J Am Assoc Gynecol Laparosc. 1996;3(4):623–5.
44. Chithra S, Manchanda R, Jain N, Lekhi A. Role of hysteroscopy in diagnosis of Asherman's syndrome. Int J Curr Res. 2016;8(05):31963–70.
45. AAGL Elevating Gynecologic Surgery. AAGL practice report: practice guidelines on intrauterine adhesions developed in collaboration with the European Society of Gynaecological Endoscopy (ESGE). Gynecol Surg. 2017;14:6. https://doi.org/10.1186/s10397-017-1007-3.

Organic Tissue Grafts Following Intrauterine Adhesiolysis

12

Mohammed Amer and Mounir Mostafa

After primary hysteroscopic adhesiolysis, the reformation of new adhesions is very frequent. The recurrence rate is related to the grade of adherences ranging from 20% to 40% [1].

The management of Asherman syndrome and intrauterine adhesions not only is limited to mechanical adhesiolysis and restoring the shape of the uterine cavity shape, but also extends to preventing the recurrence of these adhesions and enhancing the endometrial growth along the cavity inner surface [2].

Because the molecular mechanisms leading to the formation of fibrosis were poorly understood, most surgeons had to use an intrauterine device and follow treatment with high doses of sequential estrogen and progesterone to promote endometrial healing. But the inefficiency of IUDs in many reports and the side effects of systemic hormonal administration enforced more research for newer treatment options.

Biological barriers have many advantages; they can inhibit inflammatory reactions, are involved in multiple metabolic functions, and contain different kinds of growth factors [3].

In this chapter, the different modalities of intrauterine organic tissue grafts post-Asherman repair are presented. They include the use of stem cells, platelet-rich plasma, and amniotic membrane graft (Fig. 12.1).

There are no large randomized control trials or solid evidence yet that one or more of these techniques is a standard practice.

M. Amer · M. Mostafa (✉)
Obstetrics and Gynecology, Ain Shams University, Cairo, Egypt

R. Manchanda (ed.), *Intra Uterine Adhesions*,
https://doi.org/10.1007/978-981-33-4145-6_12

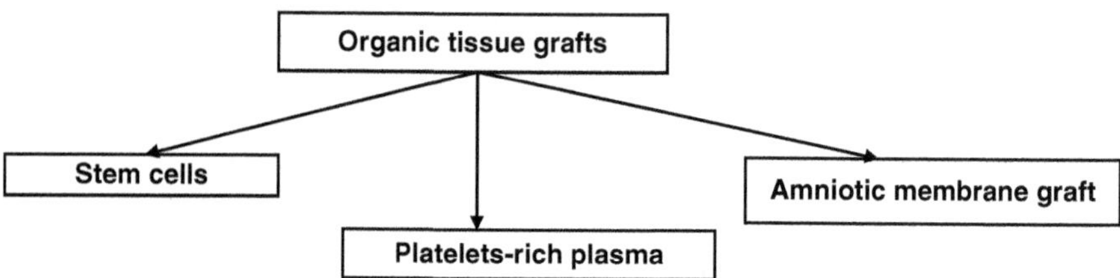

Fig. 12.1 Organic tissue grafts

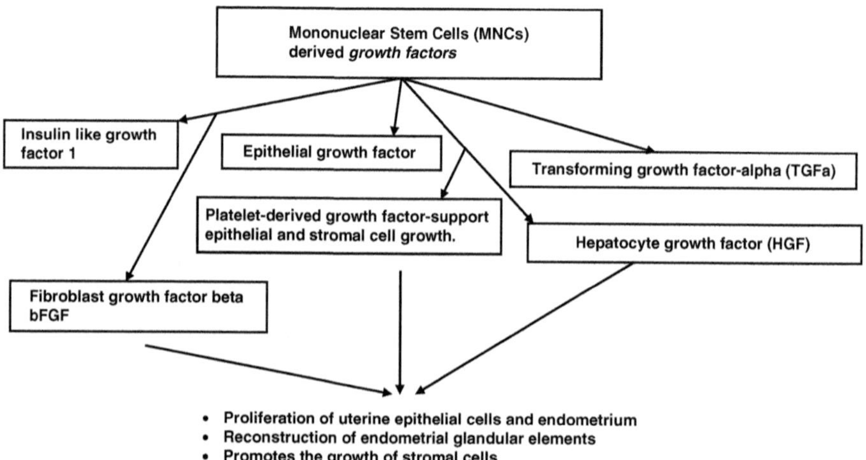

Fig. 12.2 Mononuclear stem cell (MNC)-derived *growth factors*

12.1 Stem Cells

It has been proved that bone marrow-derived stem cells travel to distant organs and contribute to tissue repair and regeneration. Stem cells have been detected in normal healthy endometrium, suggesting their role as a source of reparative cells for the endometrium [4].

Stem cells exert their therapeutic benefits mainly through the secretion of growth factors and other proteins/molecules (Fig. 12.2).

Most of the trials on intrauterine stem cells for intrauterine adhesions were done on experimental lab animals (mice). These involved the extraction of stem cells from another experimental animal, and infusing it into uterine cavity. Only few human trials are available in literature, and they involved limited sample size.

12.2 Different Procedures for Obtaining and Using the Stem Cells

1. Extraction of the endometrial angiogenic stem cells from bone marrow using complicated laboratory procedures and then distilling them directly into uterine cavity or injecting them into the subendometrial area.
2. Isolating $CD133^+$ cells through peripheral blood apheresis and delivering them into the spiral arterioles by catheterization.
3. Autologous menstrual blood-derived stromal cell transplantation into uterine cavity.

All of these trails reported endometrial thickness improvement in most of the cases, along with occurrence of normal menstruation and even conception.

12.3 Evidences

- Neeta Singh et al. [5] studied autologous bone marrow-derived stem cell implantation in the subendometrial zone followed by exogenous oral estrogen therapy, in six cases of refractory AS with failed standard treatment option of hysteroscopic adhesiolysis. Endometrial thickness (ET) was assessed at 3, 6, and 9 months. Mean of ET (mm) at 3 months (4.05 ± 1.40), 6 months (5.46 ± 1.36), and 9 months (5.48 ± 1.14) was significantly ($P < 0.05$) increased from pretreatment level (1.38 ± 0.39). Five out of six patients resumed menstruation. They concluded that the autologous stem cell implantation leads to endometrial regeneration reflected by restoration of menstruation in five out of six cases. Autologous stem cell implantation is a promising novel cell-based therapy for refractory AS.

12.3.1 Procedure

Under strict aseptic precaution, BM (30 mL) was aspirated from iliac crest using disposable BM aspiration needle (Jamshidi, 11 G) and collected in heparinized syringes. Samples were immediately transported to stem cell facility in plastic tubes for adult stem cell harvesting.

12.3.1.1 Preparation of Hematopoietic Stem Cell

The isolation of mononuclear cells (MNCs) was done by Ficoll density separation method. BM was diluted in a 1:3 ratio with ×1 phosphate-buffered saline (PBS) and layered over lymphocyte separation medium and centrifuged at a speed of 800 G for 25 min. MNC (buffy coat) was aspirated with 10 mL disposable pipette and washed thrice in heparinized normal saline (NS)/PBS to remove the traces of Ficoll. All the procedures were performed in the stem cell laboratory. Finally, MNCs were suspended in 3 mL heparinized NS.

12.3.1.2 Harvested MNC Evaluated for

- Viability: Trypan blue dye exclusion test was done to know the percentage of live cells.
- Cell morphology: MNCs were stained with Giemsa stain and observed under microscope.
- $CD34^+$ counts: MNCs were tagged with CD34 antibodies and assessed by flow cytometry to evaluate the hematopoietic stem cells.
- Total cell count: Cell numbers were assessed by counting the cell in the Neubauer chamber under microscope.

Same day the patients were taken up for stem cell implantation under intravenous (IV) sedation and antibiotic cover. The patient was laid in lithotomy position. A transvaginal probe was covered with sterile disposable probe cover with a guide attached to it. After locating the subendometrial zone on ultrasound ovum pickup needle (Cook No. 17) introduced vaginally via the lateral fornix, stem cells were implanted in the subendometrial zone transmyometrially. A volume of 3 mL of MNC was delivered at 2–3 sites (fundus, anterior, and posterior part) of the myometrium.

12.3.2 Post-procedure Care

Patients were continued on antibiotics for 5 days and started on oral estradiol valerate (Progynova), tablets 6 mg/day in three divided doses, the same day for 12 weeks, and medroxyprogesterone was given in the last 10 days.

Women who were previously amenorrheic started having cyclical bleeding after the procedure; this was taken as a sign of endometrial regeneration and was further confirmed by TVS.

Patients who started menstruation were shifted to cyclical oral estrogen (estradiol valerate) 2 mg thrice daily for 21 days (day 1 to day 26) and oral progesterone (medroxyprogesterone) 10 mg once daily from day 16 to day 25.

Santamaria et al. [6] studied the role of autologous peripheral blood $CD133^+$ bone marrow-derived stem cells (BMDSCs) for 11 patients with refractory Asherman's syndrome (AS) and/or endometrial atrophy (EA) and a wish to conceive and reported that all patients exhibited an improved uterine cavity 2 months after stem cell therapy.Endometrial thickness increased from an average of 4.3 mm (range 2.7–5) to 6.7 mm (range 3.1–12) ($P = 0.004$). Similarly, four of the five EA patients experienced an improved endometrial cavity, and endometrial thickness increased from 4.2 mm (range 2.7–5) to 5.7 mm (range 5–12) ($P = 0.03$). The beneficial effects of the cell therapy increased the mature vessel density and the duration and intensity of menses in the first 3 months, with a return to the initial levels 6 months after the treatment. Three patients became pregnant spontaneously, resulting in one baby boy born, one ongoing pregnancy, and a miscarriage. Furthermore, 7 pregnancies were obtained after 14 embryo transfers, resulting in BMDSC.

12.3.3 Procedure

Mobilization and isolation: Mobilization of BMDSCs was induced by pharmacological administration of granulocyte-colony-stimulating factor (G-CSF) (10 mg/kg/day on days −4, −3, −2, and −1).

5 Days after injection, isolation of mononuclear cells was performed by apheresis through peripheral venous access using the CobeSpectra separator (Terumo BCT, Lakewood, CO, USA) according to the manufacturer's instructions. Once the volume was adjusted to 95 g, the mononuclear antibody was added to perform $CD133^+$ cell selection and isolation using the cell sorter CliniMACS (Miltenyi Biotec GmbH, Bergisch Gladbach (Germany)), no later than 24 h after extracting mononuclear cells.

Two blood volumes were processed unless the patient showed a suboptimal mobilization of $CD133^+$ circulating cells (30/mL), in which case three blood volumes were processed. A unit of blood volume is equal to 10 L. The mean amount of mobilized volume corresponds to 26 + 2.09 L. All procedures are performed in a room with HEPA filters and controlled temperature at 22–24 °C.

The minimum of $CD133^+$ cells to be obtained by selection was 50 million cells. Isolated $CD133^+$ cells were diluted into 15–30 cm^3 of saline solution and transported in a sterile syringe to the radiology department for delivery into spiral arterioles.

12.3.4 Delivery of BMDSCs After Successful $CD133^+$ Isolation

Cell delivery to the endometrial stem cell niche via intra-arterial catheterization is performed using common femoral artery using the Seldinger technique in which a 4 F introducer allows catheterization of both hypogastric arteries with an angiographic catheter curve and a guide Terumo 0.035 in. Through the latter catheter, a 2.5 F microcatheter with a guide (0.014 in) was introduced to catheterize the uterine artery to the most distal spiral arterioles that the microcatheter could reach. Once the catheter position was stabilized and verified, 15 cm^3 of a saline suspension of the selected $CD133^+$ cells (containing 42–200 × 10^6 cells, mean 123.56 × 10^6) was injected through each uterine artery into the spiral arterioles. All patients were given HRT before and after receiving cell therapy.

Jichun Tan et al. [7] studied autologous transplantation of menstrual blood-derived stromal cells (menSCs) for regeneration of endometrium, to support pregnancy in seven patients with severe Asherman's syndrome, and reported that the ET was significantly ($P = 0.0002$) increased to 7 mm in five women, which ensured embryo implantation. Four patients underwent FET and two of them conceived successfully. One patient had spontaneous pregnancy after second menSC transplantation.

12.3.5 Procedure

Menstrual blood samples were collected by catheter rinsed by penicillin/streptomycin from patients on day 2 of their menses. The samples were transferred to phosphate-buffered saline (PBS) containing penicillin/streptomycin and heparin. Mononuclear cells were fractionated in Ficoll and cultured in Dulbecco's modified Eagle medium: nutrient mixture F-12 (Ham's) supplemented with 10% autologous serum (isolated from her own peripheral blood), 2 mM L-glutamine (HyClone), 100 U/mL penicillin, and 100 mg/mL streptomycin (HyClone).

The culture medium was changed every 3–5 days, and the cells were passaged by trypsin digestion after reaching 80–90% confluence. The culture supernatant of the menSCs was collected when the medium was changed twice and sent to the clinical laboratory for testing of bacteria, fungi, lipopolysaccharides, and hepatitis virus. The cells were abandoned upon detection of microbial contamination. The cells were cultured for about 14 days. MenSCs were transplanted before the third passage. Flow cytometry was performed to identify the phenotype of menSCs on the day immediately before transplantation. FITC-conjugated anti-human antibodies for CD34, CD44, CD45, CD90, and CD105 as well as phycoerythrin-conjugated anti-human antibodies for CD38, CD73, and SSEA-4 were used to characterize menSCs. Stained cells were analyzed with a FACScaliburTM Flow Cytometer. Autologous menSC transplantation was done on day 16 of the same menstrual cycle. MenSCs were trypsinized, washed twice, counted, and finally resuspended in sterile PBS at a concentration of 2×10^6 cells/mL.

The patients were held in a lithotomy position. A mild scratch of the endometrium was done before transplantation. Then, a transvaginal probe was inserted into the cervix guided by transabdominal B ultrasound. An internal cannula (Frydman classic catheter 4.5; Laboratoire CCD, France), filled with 0.5 mL menSC suspension, was delivered through the cervix to the fundus of the uterus to instill the menSCs. The internal tube followed by the external probe was withdrawn gently and slowly after 5 min. The patient was discharged after 2 h. The next round of cell therapy was conducted after three or more menstrual cycles if the endometrial growth was unsatisfactory.

HRT was given to stimulate endometrial growth. After day 5 of menstrual blood collection, patients were administered oral estradiol valerate tablets of 4 mg daily for 14 days. After menSC transplantation, the patients were treated with oral estradiol valerate tablets of 6 mg daily for 21 days. If the endometrium thickness was <7 mm, an intramuscular injection of 40 mg progesterone was used.

12.3.6 Stem Cells in Short

The main disadvantage of using stem cells is the high cost and complexity of the isolation process.

There are no recommendations for using stem cell therapy in uterine pathologies for except for research purposes, until future reveals the real potential of such procedures.

12.4 Platelet-Rich Plasma

Platelet-rich plasma (PRP) is plasma with at least twice the platelet concentration of normal plasma and is usually created by centrifugation filtration of autologous anti-coagulated blood.

PRP has a role in a wide range of medical applications like musculoskeletal and integumentary disease. Current management of AS should ideally be directed not only towards removal of adhesions and prevention of their re-formation, but also towards the regeneration/revival of endometrial lining in order to provide a healthy layer of cells to support the pregnancy. PRP contains many adhesive proteins (Fig. 12.3).

The introduction of PRP in the management of intrauterine lesions is very recent and a lot of trials are ongoing, to understand the real effect of PRP on endometrial growth. PRP is used to promote endometrial growth and improve pregnancy outcome during in vitro fertilization and more recently many researches showed improved outcomes after PRP usage after adhesiolysis.

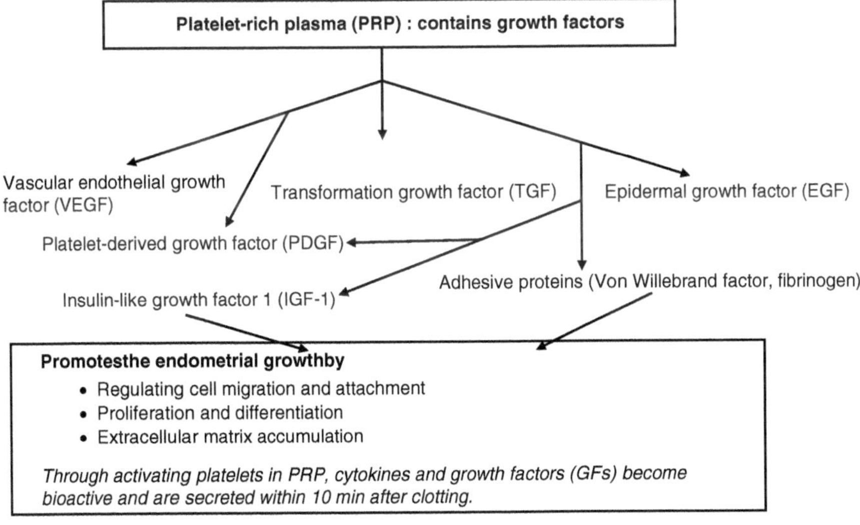

Fig. 12.3 Platelet-rich plasma (PRP): contains growth factors

Multiple methods have been developed for PRP preparation, with variation in the speed and timing of centrifugation. Platelets have to be activated as this might influence the availability of bioactive molecules and therefore tissue healing. Activation is usually done by adding calcium derivatives or thrombin (e.g., 10% $CaCl_2$) (Fig. 12.4a–d).

Half to one milliliter of PRP is then infused into the uterine cavity after the adhesiolysis and/or on subsequent occasions using a regular IUI catheter. Other alternatives include subendometrial injection of PRP by a needle under hysteroscopic guide with Cook needle or cystoscopic needle (Fig. 12.5a, b) to allow longer action of PRP, but there is no data about the superiority of this technique over simple infusion into cavity.

- Available trials and case reports have proved its efficiency in the improvement of menses and decrease in adhesion recurrence rate.
- PRP is the easiest and most practical compared to stem cells and amniotic membrane. It is also very safe and can be prepared and administered in office settings.

12.5 Evidences

Yajie Chang et al. [8] evaluated the effectiveness of PRP in the therapy of five infertile women with thin endometrium (≤7 mm) and reported successful endometrial expansion and pregnancy in all the patients after PRP infusion.

HRT protocol and PRP preparation: Estradiol valerate (Progynova; Bayer Schering Pharma, France) at 12 mg/day was given on day 3 of menstrual cycle. On the 10th day of HRT cycle, 15 mL of venous blood was drawn from the syringe

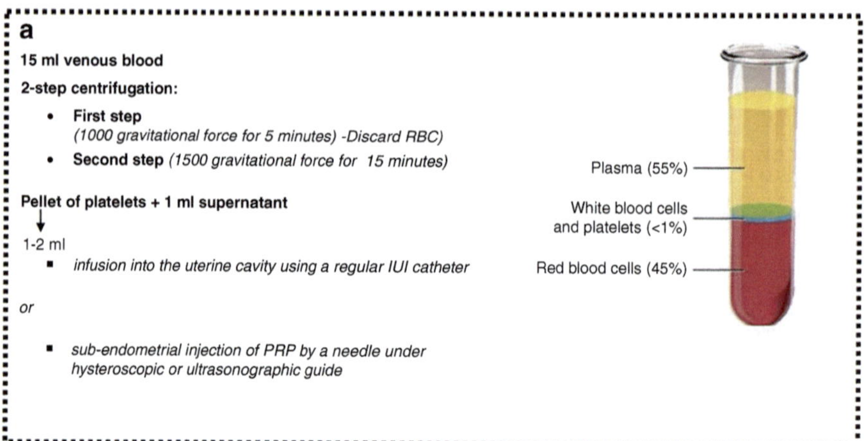

Fig. 12.4 (**a**) PRP preparation and procedure. (**b**) Dense adhesions involving >2/3rd cavity. (**c**) Adhesiolysis using scissors. (**c**) PRP containing Cook needle introduced hysteroscopically. (**d**) Subendometrial injections of PRP using Cook needle no. 17

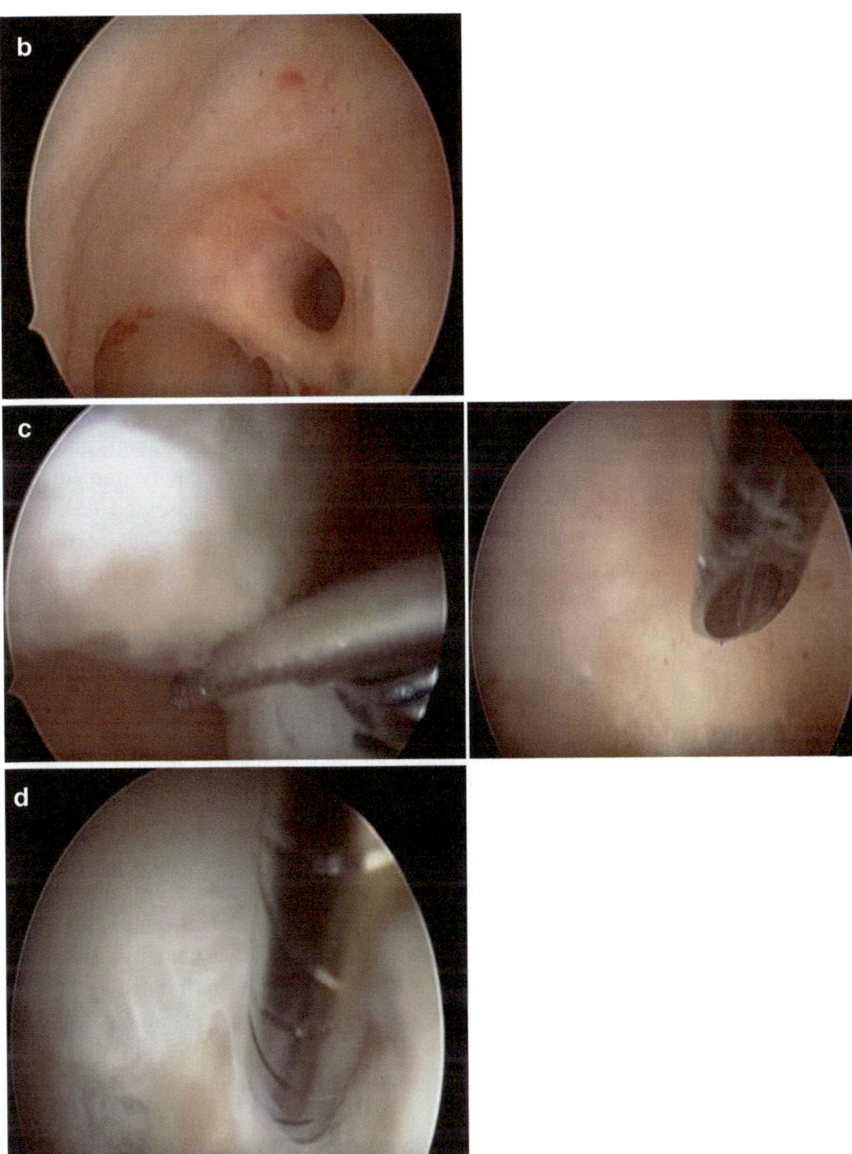

Fig. 12.4 (continued)

pre-filled with 5 mL of anticoagulant solution (ACD-A), and centrifuged immediately at 200* g for 10 min.

The blood was divided into three layers: red blood cells at the bottom, cellular plasma in the supernatant, and a buffy coat layer between them. The plasma layer and buffy coat were collected to another tube and recentrifuged at 500* g for 10 min.

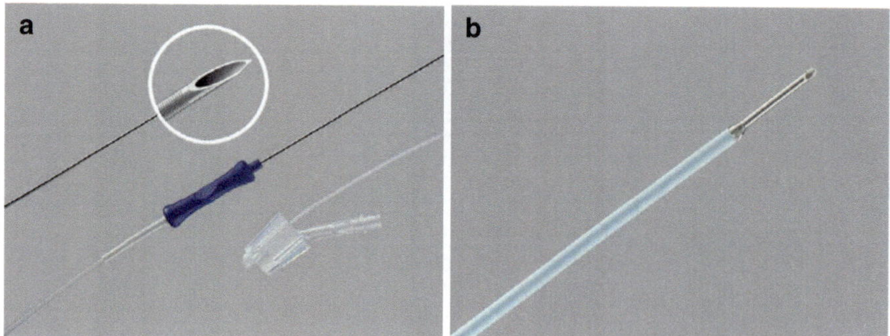

Fig. 12.5 (**a**) Cook needle. (**b**) Cystoscopic needle

The resulting pellet of platelets was mixed with 1 mL of supernatant, and then 0.5–1 mL of PRP was obtained. It was infused into the uterus cavity immediately with Tomcat catheter (0.5–1 mL). Endometrial thickness was reassessed 72 h later. If the endometrial thickness was not satisfactory, infusion of PRP was performed 1–2 times. Of five patients, only patient 2 received a single infusion, and the remaining 4 underwent 2 infusions.

Mohamed Ibrahim et al. [9] conduced a study aimed at assessment of the efficacy of the use of platelet-rich plasma (PRP) in decreasing occurrence and recurrence of intrauterine adhesions after operative hysteroscopy. 60 patients sought for conception with a history of primary or secondary infertility with severe intrauterine adhesions. 30 patients (case) were injected with PRP and 30 patients (control) with IU balloon. They reported a significant increase of menses duration among the PRP group postoperative (3.0 ± 1.2) days and preoperative menses duration (1.4 ± 1.5) days compared to balloon postoperative (1.8 ± 1.3) and preoperative (1.3 ± 1.4) days. Conclusion: Platelet-rich plasma had high efficacy and safety in terms of improvement of menses duration, amount and adhesion score in cases of sever intrauterine adhesions, and decrease in postoperative adhesion.L. Aghajanova et al. [10] studied the role of intrauterine infusion of autologous platelet-rich plasma (PRP) in the management of moderate-severe AS, particularly those resistant to standard therapies, and concluded that PRP was well tolerated and resulted in significant EMT increase after PRP infusion combined with standard surgical and medical AS treatment.

Twelve women with moderate-severe AS were recruited ($n = 5$ in control and $n = 7$ in PRP group). Endometrial thickness (EMT) and menstrual bleeding pattern were assessed before and 2 weeks after the therapy. Intrauterine adhesion and pain scores were recorded. At the end of hysteroscopy 0.5–1 mL of PRP was infused into the uterus via a Wallace catheter, followed by estrogen therapy. Control patients received an infusion of normal saline.

There was no difference in the mean age, gravity/parity, preoperative assessment of menses, mean AS hysteroscopy score (5.3 vs. 5.6), and number of patients with intrauterine balloon placement between groups. There was no difference in baseline EMT (4.92 ± 1.65 mm in PRP vs. 4.92 ± 1.2 mm in control group, $p = 0.5$). There was a significant increase in EMT after PRP infusion (7.11 ± 2.5 mm, $p = 0.044$) which was not noted in the control group (6.85 ± 3.39 mm, $p = 0.17$). Patients tolerated the procedure well (pain score 0–1/10 in PRP group), with no adverse effects. In the PRP group, there were three intrauterine pregnancies (IUP)—one after fresh embryo transfer, one after frozen embryo transfer (FET), and one after timed intercourse, long with one failed FET, one failed IUI, one pending pregnancy test after FET, and one planned FET. In the controls, there were two IUP after FET, one failed FET and two patients not pregnant after multiple rounds of timed intercourse.

The removal of scar tissue and exposure of the normal endometrial cells to the growth factors and cytokines in PRP help boost the existing cellular functions involved in tissue regeneration.

12.6 Amniotic Membrane

The amniotic membrane consisted of an epithelial monolayer on a basement membrane with an underlying collagen matrix with a few fibroblasts [11, 12].

Placing a piece of an amniotic membrane (extracted from productions of conception) at the time of hysteroscopic treatment for Asherman's syndrome is also a relatively new idea that has acquired little attention in literature [13].

12.6.1 Mechanism of Action

Amniotic membrane contains epidermal growth factor, fibroblast growth factor, and platelet-derived growth factor that may help the recovery of the injured endometrium. It also helps in epithelial cell migration and growth of the endometrium [11–15].

12.6.2 Procedure

Amnion is obtained after delivery, is simply prepared, and is cheap and no ethical issues are involved. Amniotic membrane is bluntly separated from fresh placenta after cesarean section (from consented volunteers) under aseptic conditions, and washed many times with saline. After that it is soaked in an antibiotic (e.g., cefuroxime). Amnion can be then used within a couple of hours or stored in saline and antibiotic at 4 °C up to 1 week.

Alternatives to fresh amnion include cryopreserved amniotic membrane products like amnio graft used in ocular surgeries.

After the hysteroscopic adhesiolysis, the amniotic membrane is then applied on an intrauterine balloon (or Foley's catheter) with the chorion side (mesenchymal side) of the amnion looking outside, inserted in uterus under the guidance of trans-abdominal ultrasonography, and fixed in the uterine cavity for 5 days to 2 weeks under antibiotic cover.

Most trials and meta-analyses in the literature show an increase in menstrual blood volume, but this treatment showed little effect on the rates of intrauterine adhesion recurrence.

Key Points

1. There are no large randomized control trials or solid evidence yet that one or more of these techniques is a standard practice.
2. Stem cells exert their therapeutic benefits mainly through the secretion of growth factors and other protein/molecules.
3. Stem cells can be obtained by bone marrow, peripheral blood aphaeresis, and autologous menstrual blood.
4. Platelet-rich plasma (PRP) is plasma with at least twice the platelet concentration of normal plasma and is usually created by centrifugation filtration of autologous anticoagulated blood.
5. PRP contains many adhesive proteins.
6. PRP can be infused into the uterine cavity using a regular IUI catheter or subendometrial injection by a needle under hysteroscopic or ultrasonographic guide.
7. The amniotic membrane consisted of an epithelial monolayer on a basement membrane with an underlying collagen matrix with a few fibroblasts.
8. After the hysteroscopic adhesiolysis, the amniotic membrane is then applied on an intrauterine balloon or Foley's catheter.

References

1. Hanstede MM, van der Meij E, Goedemans L, Emanuel MH, et al. Fertil Steril. 2015;104(6):1561-8.e1.
2. Dreisler E, Kjer JJ. Asherman's syndrome: current perspectives on diagnosis and management. Int J Women's Health. 2019;11:191–8.
3. Gan L, Duan H, Xu Q, et al. Human amniotic mesenchymal stromal cell transplantation improves endometrial regeneration in rodent models of intrauterine adhesions. Cytotherapy. 2017;19(5):603–16.
4. Kilic S, Yuksel B, Pinarli F, et al. Effect of stem cell application on Asherman syndrome, an experimental rat model. J Assist Reprod Genet. 2014;31(8):975–82.
5. Singh N, Mohanty S, Shankar M, Bhaskaran S, Dharmendra S. Autologous stem cell transplantation in refractory Asherman's syndrome: a novel cell based therapy. J Human Reproduct Sci. 2014;7(2):93–8. https://doi.org/10.4103/0974-1208.138864.
6. Santamaria X, Cabanillas S, Cervelló I, et al. Autologous cell therapy with CD133+ bone marrow-derived stem cells for refractory Asherman's syndrome and endometrial atrophy: a pilot cohort study. Hum Reprod. 2016;31(5):1087–96.

7. Tan J, Li P, Wang Q, et al. Autologous menstrual blood-derived stromal cells transplantation for severe Asherman's syndrome. Hum Reprod. 2016;31(12):2723–9.
8. Chang Y, Li J, Chen Y, et al. Autologous platelet-rich plasma promotes endometrial growth and improves pregnancy outcome during in vitro fertilization. Int J Clin Exp Med. 2015;8:1286–90.
9. Amer MIM, Ahmed ME-S, Kamal RM, Torky AMMAE. Value of using platelet rich plasma after hysteroscopic analysis of severe intrauterine adhesions (a randomized controlled trial). Egypt J Hosp Med. 2018;71(4):2869–74. https://doi.org/10.12816/0046137.
10. Aghajanova L, Letourneau J, Cedars MI, Huddleston HG. Autologous platelet rich plasma as a novel treatment for Asherman syndrome: results of a pilot randomized clinical trial. Fertil Steril. 2018;109(3):e1.3.
11. Domnina A, Novikova P, Obidina J, et al. Human mesenchymal stem cells in spheroids improve fertility in model animals with damaged endometrium. Stem Cell Res Ther. 2018;9(1):50.
12. Rennie K, Gruslin A, Hengstschlager M, et al. Applications of amniotic membrane and fluid in stem cell biology and regenerative medicine. Stem Cells Int. 2012;2012:721538.
13. Amer MI, Abd-El-Maeboud KH. Amnion graft following hysteroscopic lysis of intrauterine adhesions. J Obstet Gynaecol Res. 2006;32:559–66.
14. Amer MI, Abd-El-Maeboud KH, Abdelfatah I, et al. Human amnion as a temporary biologic barrier after hysteroscopic lysis of severe intrauterine adhesions: pilot study. J Minim Invasive Gynecol. 2010;17:605–11.
15. Zheng F, Zhu B, Liu Y, Wang R, Cui Y. Meta-analysis of the use of amniotic membrane to prevent recurrence of intrauterine adhesion after hysteroscopic adhesiolysis. Int J Gynaecol Obstet. 2018;143(2):145–9.

Follow-Up and Relook Hysteroscopy 13

Attilio Di Spiezio Sardo, Maria Chiara De Angelis,
Antonella D'Apolito, Jose Carugno, and Gloria Calagna

One of the main challenging issues in gynecologic practice is the high rate of adhesion re-formation after initial treatment in patients with Asherman's syndrome (AS). The incidence has been increasing over the last few decades, with a reported recurrence rate of up to 30% (1/3 with mild-to-moderate adhesions, and 2/3 with severe adhesions) likely due to an increase in iatrogenic endometrial trauma [1].

Hysteroscopic techniques have improved over the years and have allowed direct visualization of the uterine cavity. It has revolutionized the approach to the management of intrauterine adhesions (IUA), becoming the gold standard approach for the diagnosis, treatment, and follow-up of this challenging condition (Fig. 13.1). The aim of the therapeutic approach is to re-establish a pear-like-shaped uterine cavity and therefore its physiological function, facilitating communication between the endometrial cavity and both the cervical canal and the fallopian tubes. On the other hand, it is important to establish a well-defined postoperative management, focused on reducing the risk of adhesion re-formation.

Complete resolution of intrauterine adhesions is not always possible with a single procedure, especially in severe stages. For this reason, most treatment protocols include a follow-up hysteroscopy evaluation of the uterine cavity to assess endometrial restoration after the initial surgery. If this is not done, an increased obstetric risk could be observed. Therefore, it seems imperative to define the appropriate

A. D. S. Sardo (✉) · M. C. De Angelis · A. D'Apolito
Department of Public Health, School of Medicine, University of Naples Federico II, Naples, Italy

J. Carugno
Obstetrics, Gynecology and Reproductive Sciences Department, Minimally Invasive Gynecology Unit, University of Miami, Miller School of Medicine, Miami, FL, USA

G. Calagna
Obstetrics and Gynecology Unit, "Villa Sofia Cervello" Hospital, University of Palermo, Palermo, Italy

R. Manchanda (ed.), *Intra Uterine Adhesions*,
https://doi.org/10.1007/978-981-33-4145-6_13

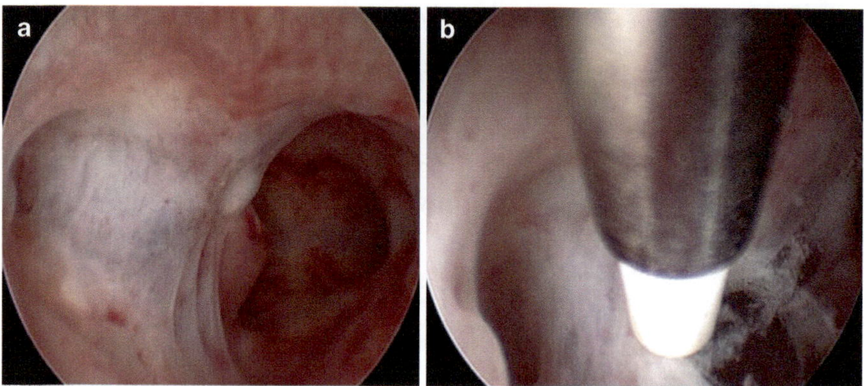

Fig. 13.1 (**a**, **b**) Adhesiolysis of moderate-to-severe intrauterine synechiae of marginal type using a 5-Fr bipolar electrode

follow-up strategy for the postoperative management of patients undergoing treatment of intrauterine adhesions.

It is important to distinguish and classify the IUA as primary when forming "ex novo," and as secondary when recurring at sites where adhesiolysis had been previously performed [2, 3]. Secondary adhesions are frequently reported in patients with a history of gynecologic procedures both for diagnostic and therapeutic purposes, or with an intracavitary trauma precipitating scar formation in the endometrium and its basal membrane, resulting in approximation and subsequent fusion of surfaces of opposite uterine walls [4, 5].

IUAs are a relevant, often unavoidable, short- or long-term consequence of hysteroscopic surgery, and the frequency with which they develop depends mainly on the type of surgical procedure, being particularly high in case of metroplasty, myomectomy, and endometrial ablation [4, 6].

Moreover, it is difficult to assess the impact of an individual intervention on the recurrence of intrauterine adhesions, as several modalities are often used in combination, and there are no much data comparing the different available treatment options. Consequently, there is no consensus on postoperative management of patients with AS.

Good surgical practice and technique are considered the "key points" for avoiding the development of IUA after hysteroscopic adhesiolysis:

- The scarred area should be resected up to the healthy myometrium providing a clean and healthy healing plane [5, 7].
- In the presence of a hard and dense adhesive area, a circular block resection should be performed (ideally under ultrasound guidance), freeing the midcavitary adhesions.
- In the event that the access to the uterine cornual area and the identification of the fallopian tubal ostia are not possible, following the balloon dilatation of the cavity, an ultrasound guide *spirotome* insertion can be used to obtain access to the cornua.

- It is important to highlight the type of energy used during the procedure. Retrospective study conducted by Mazzon et al. [8] found a very low frequency of IUA after myomectomy when using a combination of monopolar energy and cold knife resection [8]. In a retrospective case series, Touboul et al. [9] determined the rate of uterine synechiae after bipolar hysteroscopic myomectomy among fertile patients and found that using bipolar energy to perform the resection is associated with lower IUA recurrence rate compared to monopolar energy, but randomized controlled trials to evaluate this fact are still needed [9]. Another advantage of using bipolar energy is that this system requires no cervical dilatation, does not require the use of dispersive return electrodes, nor generates stray currents, therefore minimizing complications and decreasing the possibility of adhesion re-formation (Fig. 13.2).

It should also be noted that dilatation of the cervical canal in AS can be especially difficult due to the fact that IUAs can be often associated with fibrosis at the internal or external cervical os which leads to higher risk of uterine perforation. Novel mini-resectoscope with a smaller scope diameter (5 mm), requiring minimal

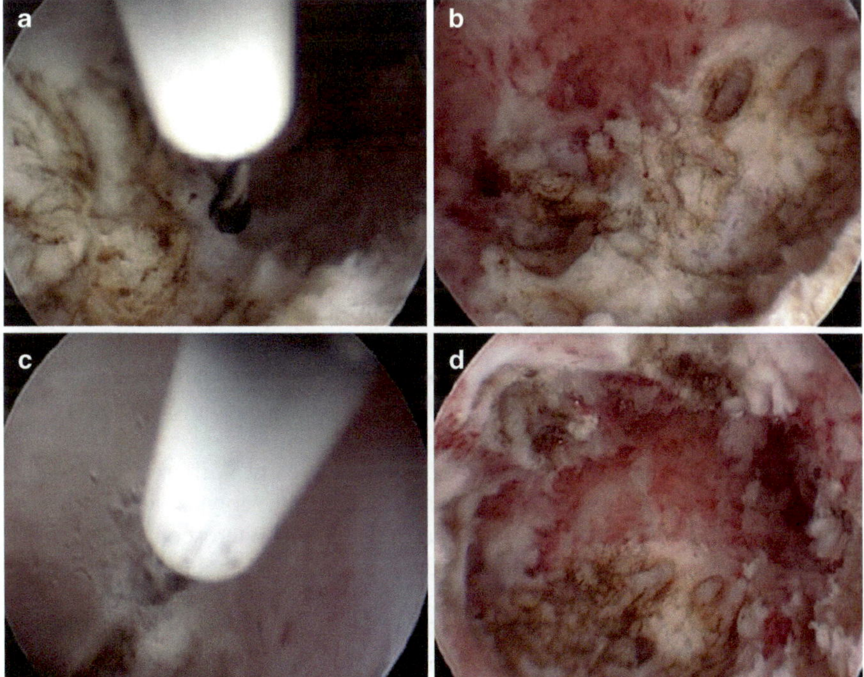

Fig. 13.2 (**a**–**d**) Treatment of Asherman's syndrome with a 5-Fr bipolar electrode. First, the fibrous patches protruding into the cavity are removed (**a**, **b**); then multiple longitudinal incisions (about 4 mm in depth) are made on the fibrotic tissue overlying the uterine wall (**c**), starting from the fundus and proceeding as far as the isthmic region. Hysteroscopic intracavitary view upon completion of the procedure (**d**)

cervical dilatation, is the ideal device for hysteroscopic adhesiolysis, reducing the chance of cervical trauma, both for preventing adhesion re-formation and reducing operative morbidity.

Different strategies have been proposed to prevent the recurrence of adhesions after surgery but no consensus regarding the optimal method has yet been defined, due to the poor quality of evidence in the literature.

Recent literature data emphasize the role of "relook" or "early second-look" hysteroscopy (usually performed a few days after surgery) after many intracavitary procedures, being particularly recommended in cases of severe Asherman's syndrome.

As a matter of fact, complete resolution of adhesions is not always possible with a single procedure, especially in severe stages, where a high recurrence rate is documented. Timely recognition of recurrence of adhesions is essential to provide the best outcome; therefore it may be needed to perform a second surgery [10]. For this reason, most treatment protocols include a follow-up hysteroscopic procedure to assess endometrial restoration after the initial surgery.

Currently, there is no clear consensus on how to perform the follow-up management of patients undergoing intrauterine lysis of adhesions.

13.1 Follow-Up Modalities

- Ultrasound
- Hysterosalpingography
- Second-look hysteroscopy

Ultrasound is an accurate and cost-effective tool for measuring endometrial thickness.

Hysterosalpingography has the advantage to check tubal patency also allowing to "see" thin adhesions.

Hysteroscopy remains the only method allowing direct visualization inside the uterine cavity providing an accurate estimation of adhesion recurrence and it is the most commonly used modality in clinical practice.

In a randomized study, Pabuccu et al. [11] compared two different approaches in preventing IUA re-formation after hysteroscopic adhesiolysis, to evaluate the importance of an early hysteroscopy after the initial hysteroscopic surgery for secondary prevention of postoperative IUA. Thirty-six patients (group 1) with an intrauterine device (IUD) inserted at the time of the initial hysteroscopic adhesiolysis had an early "second-look" in-office hysteroscopy 1 week later (with further adhesiolysis when needed) and a "third-look" in-office hysteroscopy 2 months later and were compared to 35 patients (group 2) who also had an IUD placed at the initial procedure, but did not undergo early second-look hysteroscopy 1 week later. Both groups underwent 2 months of the same estrogen and progestin therapy. At follow-up, the IUA formation rate was significantly lower in group 1 ($p < 0.05$) [11].

Robinson et al. [12] evaluated the role of serial office hysteroscopy performed every 1–3 weeks after hysteroscopic adhesiolysis in 24 patients. Each operative hysteroscopy was also followed by hormonal therapy (25 days of oral conjugated estrogens [2.5 mg] and 5 days of combined conjugated estrogen/medroxyprogesterone acetate [2.5/10 mg] therapy). As a result, AS improved in 92% of cases. In a recent study, Sebbag et al. [13] analyzed the prevalence of IUA development in women undergoing hysteroscopic resection of submucous myomas, polyps, and intrauterine synechiae, evaluating the efficiency of a second-look hysteroscopy to diagnose and treat postsurgical adhesions. They found that in 55.2% of cases, IUA could be treated by second-look hysteroscopy.

- ***These results therefore validate the need for performing a second-look diagnostic hysteroscopy following surgical hysteroscopies.***
- ***Although many studies now recommend very early second-look hysteroscopy, the right interval between the initial operative procedure and the second-look hysteroscopy has not been defined yet.***

Kodaman and Arici [14] proposed that if adhesions were to recur, they would be formed by the 5th postoperative day, after the time called "lag period" of wound healing.

According to Shokeir et al. [15], there is a different histological composition of the adhesions based on the time elapsed after the surgery. IUAs formed immediately after the surgery are mainly composed of grade I vs. grade II/III; indeed, early office hysteroscopy allows the lysis of newly formed adhesions, which are usually thin and filmy and easy to cut, whereas adhesions appearing a longer time after the initial operation are thick and fibrous needing more extensive surgery. Nevertheless, there is no solid evidence on how early the second-look hysteroscopy has to be performed [15].

Evidence extrapolated from laparoscopic surgery indicates that a repeat hysteroscopy within 48 h of the initial procedure is likely to facilitate the final removal of adhesion reformation. This procedure could be done without anesthesia, using the hysteroscope and the hysteroscopic grasping forceps, and all intrauterine material barrier placed at the initial procedure (i.e., hyaluronic acid gel) should be removed. Adhesions are recognized and easily lysed in this early stage. Reinsertion of an adhesion barrier such as hyaluronic acid is recommended and a final hysteroscopic evaluation is planned after the first or second menstrual period.

Frequently, the hysteroscopic second-look procedure performed within 1 month after the initial surgery, following the next menstrual cycle, seems to be an effective prophylaxis strategy for recurrent synechiae. It allows to evaluate the normalization of the uterine cavity, along with the option of immediate lysis of any small persistent synechiae.

It is important to provide an adequate follow-up after the initial hysteroscopic lysis of IUA. Traditionally, authors variably performed a "follow-up" hysteroscopy 2–4 months after the initial procedure. However, data is limited and mostly obtained from non-randomized studies with few patients limiting the available data to draw conclusions from.

As we stated at the beginning of this chapter, hysteroscopy is a simple, safe, and useful procedure for the evaluation of postsurgical IUA, both for treatment and follow-up of intrauterine pathology; then, hysteroscopy may also be useful for verifying the efficacy of anti-adhesive methods.

Over the years, different preventive adhesion measures have been studied. Barrier methods are widely used for the prevention of postoperative IUA based on the idea that the separation of endometrial layers after hysteroscopic surgery helps to prevent adhesion recurrence and could promote physiological endometrial regeneration [10]. More difficult-to-evaluate IUA prevention options are the use of intrauterine device (IUD) and hormonal and antibiotic therapy, because of their use in association with other IUA prevention strategies.

Regarding postoperative estrogen treatment, it has not yet been standardized in terms of dose, duration, route of administration, or combination with progesterone. Estrogen supplementation is commonly given postoperatively to stimulate endometrial growth, producing beneficial effects in patients with IUA undergoing adhesiolysis.

The use of anti-adhesive gels to prevent or reduce postoperative adhesion formation is generally a well-accepted practice. A higher number of randomized and non-randomized studies have shown that intrauterine use of anti-adhesive gels is an effective strategy to reduce the need for repeated interventions after hysteroscopic surgery due to postoperative IUA formation [5, 7, 16–20].

Different anti-adhesive gels have been used (described ***in detail in Chap. 11***):

1. Auto-cross-linked hyaluronic acid (ACP) gel
2. Hyaluronate–carboxymethyl cellulose membrane (CH)
3. Polyethylene oxide-sodium carboxymethyl-cellulose (POC) gel

A reduction of development of de novo post-hysteroscopic IUA and a significant decrease in adhesion severity have been observed after application of ACP gel or CH. Moreover, promising results are also related to the use of POC gel [5].

In cases where additional prevention by permanent cavity distention is necessary, it is recommended to place a device inside the uterine cavity such as a ***Word catheter:*** it combines the advantages of the IUD and Foley catheter without having their disadvantages (discomfort, as well as the risk of ascending infections). The Word catheter should be left in place for a period of 1–3 months and is removed by perforation of the balloon with the hysteroscope in an office procedure (Fig. 13.3a, b).

13.2 AAGL/ESGE 2017: Guideline for Postoperative Assessment After Treatment of Intrauterine Adhesions

Follow-up assessment of the uterine cavity after treatment of IUAs is recommended, preferably with hysteroscopy: **Level B**.

To conclude, there is a paucity of high-quality data regarding IUAs. Despite advances in hysteroscopic surgery, and various methods for prevention of recurrent

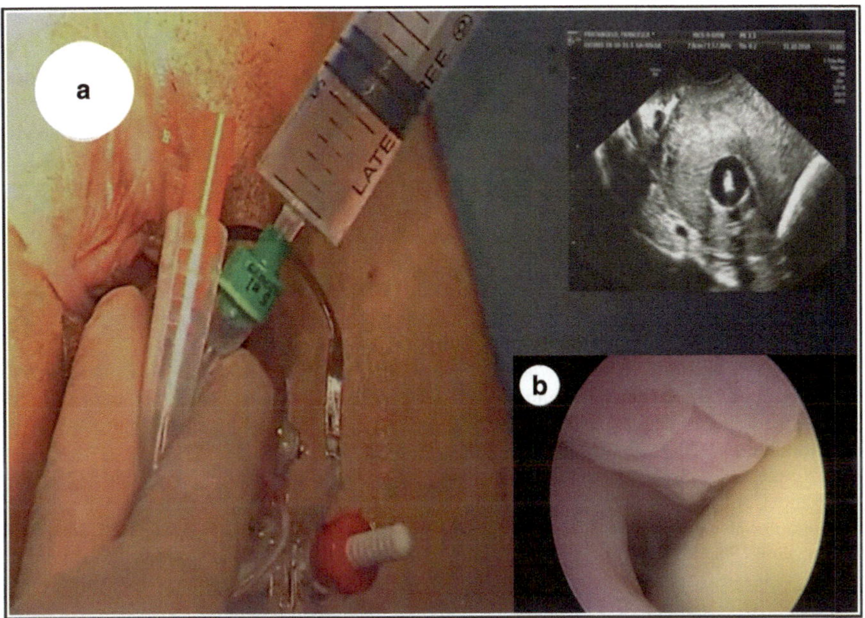

Fig. 13.3 (**a**, **b**) Insertion of a 10 French silicone balloon under ultrasound control for cavity dilatation (**a**). In **b**, hysteroscopic view of Word catheter

adhesive disease, AS recurrence rates remain high, so we must continue to investigate the ideal follow-up strategy looking for the best technique that reduces new adhesion formation. Although routine early second-look hysteroscopy could be recommended for all women undergoing extensive hysteroscopic resection, randomized prospective controlled trials are still needed to determine the optimal anti-adhesive method for routine use in all women undergoing gynecological intrauterine procedures.

Key Points

1. One of the main challenging issues in gynecologic practice is the high rate of adhesion re-formation after initial treatment in patients with Asherman's syndrome.
2. The aim of the therapeutic approach is to re-establish a pear-like-shaped uterine cavity and therefore its physiological function, facilitating communication between the endometrial cavity and both the cervical canal and the fallopian tubes.
3. Good surgical practice and technique are considered the "key points" for avoiding the development of IUA after hysteroscopic adhesiolysis:
4. Follow-up modalities are ultrasound, hysterosalpingography, and second-look hysteroscopy.
5. Follow-up assessment of the uterine cavity after treatment of IUAs is recommended, preferably with hysteroscopy.

References

1. AAMIG. AAGL practice report: practice guidelines for management of intrauterine synechiae. J Minim Invasive Gynecol. 2010;17:1–7.
2. Hellebrekers BW, Trimbos-Kemper TC, Trimbos JB, Emeis JJ, Kooistra T. Use of fibrinolytic agents in the prevention of post-operative adhesion formation. Fertil Steril. 2000;74:203–12.
3. Diamond MP, Freeman ML. Clinical implications of postsurgical adhesions. Hum Reprod Update. 2001;7:567–76.
4. Tulandi T. Introduction—prevention of adhesion formation: the journey continues. Hum Reprod Update. 2001;7(6):545–6.
5. Di Spiezio Sardo A, Calagna G, Scognamiglio M, O'Donovan P, Campo R, De Wilde RL. Prevention of intrauterine post-surgical adhesions in hysteroscopy. A systematic review. Eur J Obstet Gynecol Reprod Biol. 2016;203:182–92.
6. Guida M, Acunzo G, Di Spiezio Sardo A, Bifulco G, Piccoli R, Pellicano M, Cerrota G, Cirillo D, Nappi C. Effectiveness of auto-cross-linked hyaluronic acid gel in the prevention of intrauterine adhesions after hysteroscopic surgery: a prospective randomized, controlled study. Hum Reprod. 2004;19:1461–4.
7. Di Spiezio Sardo A, Spinelli M, Bramante S, Scognamiglio M, Greco E, Guida M, Cela V, Nappi C. Efficacy of a polyethylene oxide-sodium carboxymethylcellulose gel in prevention of intrauterine adhesions after hysteroscopic surgery. J Minim Invasive Gynecol. 2011;18:462–9.
8. Mazzon I, Favilli A, Cocco P, Grasso M, Horvath S, Bini V, Di Renzo GC, Gerli S. Does cold loop hysteroscopic myomectomy reduce intrauterine adhesions? A retrospective study. Fertil Steril. 2014;101:294–8.
9. Touboul C, Fernandez H, Deffieux X, Berry R, Frydman R, Gervaise A. Uterine synechiae after bipolar hysteroscopic resection of submucosal myomas in patients with infertility. Fertil Steril. 2009;92:1690–3.
10. Conforti A, Alviggi C, Mollo A, De Placido G, Magos A. The management of Asherman syndrome: a review of literature. Reprod Biol Endocrinol. 2013;11:118.
11. Pabuccu R, Onalan G, Kaya C, Selam B, Ceyhan T, Ornek T, Kuzudisli E. Efficiency and pregnancy outcome of serial intrauterine device-guided hysteroscopic adhesiolysis of intrauterine synechiae. Fertil Steril. 2008;90:1973–7.
12. Robinson JK, Swedarsky Colimon LM, Isaacson KB. Postoperative adhesiolysis therapy for intrauterine adhesions (Asherman's syndrome). Fertil Steril. 2008;90:409–14.
13. Sebbag L, Even M, Fay S, Carbonnel M, Revaux A, Naoura I, Ayoubi JM. Early second-look hysteroscopy: prevention and treatment of intrauterine post-surgical adhesions. Front Surg. 2019;6:50.
14. Kodaman PH, Arici A. Intra-uterine adhesions and fertility outcome: how to optimize success? Curr Opin Obstet Gynecol. 2007;19:207–14.
15. Shokeir TA, Fawzy M, Tatongy M. The nature of intrauterine adhesions following reproductive hysteroscopic surgery as determined by early and late follow-up hysteroscopy: clinical implications. Arch Gynecol Obstet. 2008;277:423–7.
16. Acunzo G, Guida M, Pellicano M, Tommaselli GA, Di Spiezio Sardo A, Bifulco G, Cirillo D, Taylor A, Nappi C. Effectiveness of auto-cross-linked hyaluronic acid gel in the prevention of intrauterine adhesions after hysteroscopic adhesiolysis: a prospective randomized, controlled study. Hum Reprod. 2003;18:1918–21.
17. Kim T, Ahn KH, Choi DS, Hwang KJ, Lee BI, Jung MH, Kim JW, Kim JH, Cha SH, Lee KH, Lee KS, Oh ST, Cho CH, Rhee JH. A randomized, multi-center, clinical trial to assess the efficacy and safety of alginate carboxymethylcellulose hyaluronic acid compared to carboxymethylcellulose hyaluronic acid to prevent postoperative intrauterine adhesion. J Minim Invasive Gynecol. 2012;19:731–6.

18. Fuchs N, Smorgick N, Ben Ami I, Vaknin Z, Tovbin Y, Halperin R, Pansky M. Intercoat (Oxiplex/AP Gel) for preventing intrauterine adhesions after operative hysteroscopy for suspected retained products of conception: double-blind, prospective, randomized pilot study. J Minim Invasive Gynecol. 2014;21:126–30.
19. Ludwin A, Ludwin I, Pitynski K, Banas T, Jach R. Role of morphologic characteristics of the uterine septum in the prediction and prevention of abnormal healing outcomes after hysteroscopic metroplasty. Hum Reprod. 2014;29:1420–31.
20. Hanstede MMF, van der Meij E, Goedemans L, Emanuel MH. Results of centralized Asherman surgery, 2003–2013. Fertil Steril. 2015;104:1561–8.

Complications and Fertility Potential Following Adhesiolysis

14

Luis Alonso Pacheco, Jose Carugno, Douglas Timmons, and Marta Garcia Sanchez

14.1 Introduction

The presence of intrauterine adhesions and the association with secondary amenorrhea were first described by Dr. Fritsh in 1894. In 1948, Dr. Joseph G. Asherman published a series of papers describing the etiology, symptoms, imaging findings, and fertility outcomes, and the condition has been known as Asherman's syndrome (AS) since. Asherman's syndrome was primarily described as an outcome of trauma to the basal layer of the endometrium, with subsequent formation of fibrotic adhesions leading to either partial or complete obstruction of the cervical canal or uterine cavity resulting in menstrual abnormalities, infertility, or recurrent pregnancy loss [1]. The initial definition of AS included confirmed IUAs with clinical features of amenorrhea, infertility, or recurrent pregnancy loss; however, today the presence of IUAs regardless of additional clinical features is often referred to as AS. For many, the terminologies Asherman's syndrome (AS), intrauterine adhesions (IUA), and intrauterine synechiae (IUS) are interchangeable.

The exact prevalence of AS is difficult to identify as a large proportion of patients have no symptoms. The last worldwide investigation found that the highest prevalence of AS has been found in Israel, Greece, and South America [2]. AS was initially described to occur following trauma to a gravid uterus. Curettage in the postpartum period, following a spontaneous abortion or during an elective

L. Alonso Pacheco (✉)
Gynecology Endoscopy Unit, Centro Gutenberg, Malaga, Spain

Unidad de Reproducción Asistida Hospital Quirónsalud, Malaga, Spain

J. Carugno · D. Timmons
Department of Obstetrics, Gynecology and Reproductive Sciences, University of Miami, Miller School of Medicine, Miami, FL, USA

M. G. Sanchez
Unidad de Reproducción Asistida Hospital Quirónsalud, Malaga, Spain

R. Manchanda (ed.), *Intra Uterine Adhesions*,
https://doi.org/10.1007/978-981-33-4145-6_14

termination of pregnancy, or following a cesarean section have all been implicated to lead to IUAs. While trauma to the gravid uterus remains the most important risk factor for the development of IUAs, trauma to a nongravid uterus, infections, uterine anomalies, and genetic predispositions have also been linked to the development of IUAs resulting in potential AS.

The presence of IUAs can vary dramatically from patient to patient. There are numerous classifications of IUAs that exist, and all require the use of hysteroscopy to determine the extent and characteristics of the adhesions. A very commonly used classification system was proposed by the American Fertility Society which classifies the severity of the disease in three stages as follows [3]:

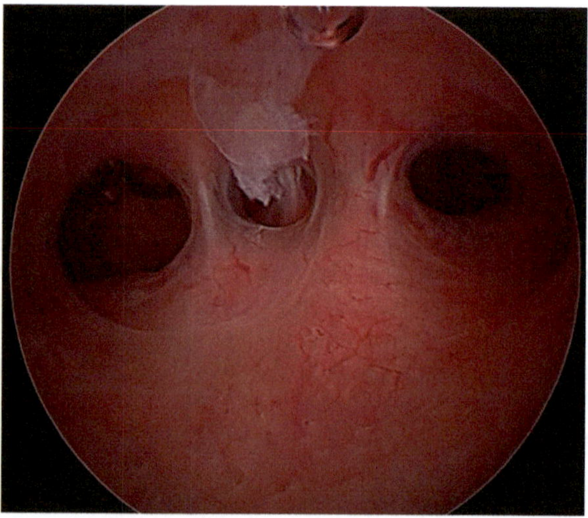

Mild disease: few filmy adhesions involving less than a third of the uterine cavity with normal menses or hypomenorrhea

Moderate disease: filmy and dense adhesions, the involvement of one-third to two-thirds of cavity and hypomenorrhea

Severe disease: dense adhesions involving more than two-thirds of the cavity with amenorrhea

Treatment of IUAs depends on the associated clinical manifestations. IUAs are not life threatening, and in the asymptomatic patient should be treated with expectant management. Surgical intervention is only indicated when patients present with signs or symptoms of pain infertility, recurrent pregnancy loss, or menstrual abnormalities including hematometra. Multiple surgical interventions have been described for the treatment of IUAs; however, hysteroscopic adhesiolysis remains the gold standard for surgical management [4]. Hysteroscopic adhesiolysis has been proven to be a very safe procedure and provides direct visualization of adhesions to increase surgical precision [5]. In cases of mild disease with thin filmy adhesions, simply distending the uterus with fluid media is enough to break the adhesions and restore normal anatomy. If more disease is encountered, adhesiolysis can be performed with hysteroscopic scissors, biopsy forceps, and monopolar or bipolar electrocautery.

14.1.1 Complications Following Adhesiolysis

Complications can be divided into intraoperative complications, and postoperative complications. As with all operative hysteroscopy, the two major intraoperative complications encountered are bleeding and perforation. The most common intraoperative complication is hemorrhage, which has been reported in 6–27% of cases [1]. Injury to myometrial blood vessels may obstruct a surgeon's view and enable for a more rapid absorption of the distention media possibly leading to major electrolyte disturbances. Uterine perforation is the second most common intraoperative complication and is seen in 2–5% of cases but has been reported in up to 9% of patients where severe IUAs were encountered. Table 14.1 includes documented complications following hysteroscopy adhesiolysis.

Surgical success at the time of surgery is typically believed to be achieved with restoration of a normal-appearing uterine cavity, which is accomplished in 57–98% of cases [6]. Despite removal of all adhesions, and restoration of a normal uterine cavity, adhesiolysis is associated with a high rate of IUA re-formation. The rate of re-formation of adhesions is high and is seen in 3.1–23.5% of cases, and has been reported in 20–62% of severe cases (Table 14.2). Numerous studies have investigated methods to decrease the re-formation of intrauterine adhesions.

Table 14.1 Complications of hysteroscopic adhesiolysis for Asherman's syndrome

Study	Year of publication	Complications	All cases	Severe cases
Valle and Sciarra	1988	Perforation	5/187 (2.7%)	3/47 (6.4%)
Pistofidis et al.	1996	Hemorrhage	5/86 (5.8%)	3/11 (27.3%)
Pabuccu et al.	1997	Perforation	1/40 (2.5%)	1/10 (10%)
McComb and Wagner	1997	Perforation	–	3/6 (50%)
		Hemorrhage	–	1/6 (16.7%)
Broome and Vancaillie	1999	Perforation	–	2/55 (3.6%)
Feng et al.	1999	Perforation	4/365 (1.1%)	4/39 (10.3%)
Capella-Allouc et al.	1999	Perforation	–	4/31 (12.9%)

Adapted from Yu et al. [1]

Table 14.2 Outcome of hysteroscopic adhesiolysis for Asherman's syndrome: restoration of menstruation in women presenting with amenorrhea or hypomenorrhea

Study	Year of publication	Normal menses following surgery, number (%)	Re-formation of intrauterine adhesions	Re-formation of intrauterine adhesions in severe cases
Fedele et al.	1986	11/21 (52.4%)	–	–
Valle and Sciarra	1988	149/169 (88.2%)	44/187 (23.5%)	23/47 (48.9%)
Pabuccu et al.	1997	29/34 (85.3%)	8/40 (20%)	6/10 (60%)
Feng et al.	1999	294/351 (83.8%)	–	–
Capella-Allouc et al.	1999	–	–	10/16 (62.5%)
Preutthipan and Linasmita	2000	45/50 (85%)	2/65 (3.1%)	2/10 (20%)

Adapted from Yu et al. [1]

Table 14.3 reports different studies investigating IUA re-formation. At this time, no consensus protocol exists to prevent the recurrence of IUAs. Patients with severe disease should be counseled at the time of initial surgery for need for possible repeat surgery, as approximately 1/3 required a repeat procedure due to IUA re-formation [7].

14.1.2 Fertility Potential Following Adhesiolysis

Secondary infertility as the initial presenting symptom has been reported in up to 45% of patients, and the pursuit of fertility is the most common indication for hysteroscopic adhesiolysis [8]. Implantation issues have been hypothesized in patients with IUAs, and hysteroscopic adhesiolysis has been shown to improve endometrial thickness and endometrial receptivity [9]. Numerous studies have been performed documenting fertility outcomes following adhesiolysis, with pregnancy rates ranging from 10.5% to 100% [10]. Guo et al. performed a meta-analysis which included 54 studies, and found an overall pregnancy rate for all subjects of 50.7% following adhesiolysis, Table 14.4. When looking at pregnancy rates before and after surgery, one study found a pregnancy rate of 65.5% after adhesiolysis, compared to only 18% preoperatively [5]. That same study found a live birth rate of 36% after adhesiolysis, compared to only 14.7% preoperatively. Most patients attempting to conceive are able to achieve a pregnancy within 1 year postoperatively, and up to 97.2% can conceive within 24 months [11, 12].

Table 14.3 Reports comparing various modalities to reduce re-formation of adhesion postresection

	Study design	Comparison groups	Relevant information	Outcomes
Solid barriers				
Orhue et al.	Prospective cohort study	IUD vs. Foley catheter	IUD arm: 51 women with Lippes loop IUD placed after surgery for 3 months Foley arm: 59 women with a Foley catheter placed postoperatively for 10 days	Absent menses: 19% in Foley group vs. 38% in IUD group ($p<0.03$) Pregnancy rate: 34% in Foley group vs. 28% in IUD group ($p=0.4656$) Fewer infections and fewer recurrent adhesions in Foley group
Lin et al.	Randomized trial	IUD vs. intrauterine balloon	IUD arm: 80 women for 1 week postsurgery Foley arm: 82 women for 1 week postsurgery	No difference in adhesion re-formation (35% in IUD vs. 30% in Foley group) No report on pregnancy outcomes
Semisolid barriers				
Acunzo et al.	Randomized trial	Hyaluronic acid gel (hyalobarrier gel; Baxter International Inc., Deerfield, IL) vs. no treatment	Hyalobarrier arm: 43 women No treatment arm: 41 women	Second-look hysteroscopy 3 months after surgery for intrauterine adhesions 14% (6/43) in hyaluronic acid arm vs. 32% (13/41) in no-treatment arm ($p < 0.05$)
Guida et al.	Randomized trial	ACP vs. no treatment	ACP arm: 67 women No-treatment arm: 65 women	Second-look hysteroscopy after surgery for intrauterine adhesions 10.4% with adhesions in the ACP arm vs. 26.2% in the no-treatment arm ($p < 0.05$)
Tsapanos et al.	Randomized trial	Modified hyaluronic acid + carboxymethylcellulose (Seprafilm; Genzyme Corp., Cambridge, MA) vs. no-treatment control	Seprafilm arm: 50 women Control arm: 100 women Data were stratified on whether or not a woman had a D&C before surgery for removal of adhesions	8 months after surgery in women who did not have a D&C: 100% (32/32) pregnant in Seprafilm arm vs. 54% (34/56) in the control arm ($p < 0.05$) If no pregnancy after 8 months all got hysterosalpingography: 10% (1/10) had intrauterine adhesions at hysterosalpingography in Seprafilm arm vs. 50% (7/14) in the control arm

(continued)

Table 14.3 (continued)

	Study design	Comparison groups	Relevant information	Outcomes
Hooker et al.	Randomized trial	ACP vs. no treatment	ACP arm: 77 women Control arm: 72 women	Second-look hysteroscopy Intrauterine adhesions in ACP arm were seen in 13% (10/77) vs. 30.6% (22/72) in the control group ($p = 0.013$)
Hormonal treatments				
Farhi et al.	Randomized trial	Hormones vs. no hormones	Hormone arm: 30 women (daily 2 mg estradiol valerate for 21 days + 0.5 mg norgestrel for 10 days) Control arm: 30 women	Hormone arm had greater endometrial thickness than control group (0.84 cm vs. 0.67 cm) ($p = 0.02$)
Mixed comparisons				
Sanfilippo et al.	Randomized trial	IUD + hormones vs. hormones only	IUD + hormone arm: 26 women Hormone-only arm: 9 women	No difference in postoperative intrauterine adhesion re-formation Pregnancy rate slightly higher in IUD + hormone group
Amer et al.	3-arm pilot randomized trial	Fresh amnion vs. dry amnion vs. intrauterine balloon	Fresh amnion arm: 15 women Dry amnion arm: 15 women Intrauterine balloon arm: 15 women	Diagnostic hysteroscopy after 2–4 months Amnion grafts reduced re-formation of adhesions ($p = 0.003$) Fresh amnion superior to dry amnion ($p = 0.01$) Of the 10 patients who were pregnant, 80% (8/10) had amnion graft and 20% (2/10) had balloon placement
Lin et al.	Retrospective cohort	Balloon catheter vs. IUD vs. hyaluronic gel vs. control	Balloon catheter arm: 20 women IUD arm: 28 women Hyaluronic gel arm: 18 women Control arm: 41 women	At second-look hysteroscopy: balloon group had the lowest number of adhesions ($p < 0.001$). IUD group had fewer adhesions than the gel and control groups

Adapted from Khan and Goldberg [8]

Table 14.4 Pregnancy rate and live birth rate following adhesiolysis

Authors	Design	Pregnancy rate	Live birth	Authors	Design	Pregnancy rate	Live birth
Forssman L, 1965	Retro	15/35 (42.9)	13/24 (54.2)	Fernandez H, 2012	Retro	9/22 (40.9)	6/9 (66.7)
Comninos AC, 1969	Retro	30/68 (44.1)	28/30 (93.3)	Myers EM, 2012	Retro	6/8 (75.0)	–
Oelsner G, 1974	–	16/41 (39.0)	14/20 (70.0)	Malhortra N, 2012	Pro	5/40 (12.5)	2/5 (40.0)
Jewelewicz R, 1976	Retro	18/34 (52.9)	10/18 (55.6)	Tuuli MG, 2012	Retro	–	–
Sugimoto O, 1978	Retro	79/192 (41.2)	47/79 (59.5)	Sendag F, 2013	Retro	4/14 (28.5)	3/4 (75.0)
Bergquist CA, 1981	Pro	19/25 (76.0)	13/19 (68.4)	Urman B, 2013	Retro	13.70%	–
Friedman A, 1986	Retro	36/33 (78.8)	23/24 (95.8)	Fuchs N, 2014	RCT	10/52 (19.2)	–
Valle RF, 1988	Retro	143/187 (76.5)	–	Ghahiry AA, 2014	Pro	6/16 (37.5)	–
Goldenberg M, 1995	Pro	20/35 (57.1)	–	SongD, 2014	Retro	20/76 (26.3)	12/20 (60.0)
Roge P, 1996	Retro	28/50 (56.0)	24/34 (70.6)	Tsui KH, 2014	Retro	4/4 (100)	2/4 (50.0)
Chen FP, 1997	Retro	3/7 (42.9)	2/3 (66.7)	Xiao SS, 2014	Retro	314/475 (66.1)	201/314 (64.0)
McComb PF, 1997	–	5/6 (83.3)	4/5 (80.0)	Bhandari S, 2015	Pro	16/60 (16.3)	10/16 (62.5)
Pabuccu R, 1997	Retro	34/40 (85.0)	23/34 (67.7)	Bougie O, 2015	Retro	6/19 (31.6)	5/6 (83.3)
Protopapas A, 1998	Pro	3/7 (42.4)	1/4 (25.0)	Kim MJ, 2015	–	8/47 (17.0)	4/8 (50.0)
Capella-Allouc S, 1999	Retro	12/28 (42.9)	9/15 (60)	Krajcovicova R, 2015	Pro	42/60 (70.0)	18/42 (42.9)
Feng ZC, 1999	Retro	156/186 (83.9)	–	Takai I, 2015	Retro	25/78 (32.1)	–
Orhue AAE, 2003	Retro	34/110 (30.9)	18/34 (52.9)	Thubert T, 2015	Retro	29/73 (39.7)	20/29 (69.0)
Zikopoulos KA, 2004	Retro	20/46 (43.5)	20/20 (100)	Sanad AS, 2016	Pro	40/61 (65.6)	22/40 (55.0)
Efetie ER, 2006	Retro	8/71 (11.3)	–	Chen L, 2017	Retro	160/332 (48.2)	137/160 (85.6)
Fernandez H, 2006	Retro	28/64 (43.8)	21/28 (75.0)	Chen Y, 2017	Pro	43/97 (44.3)	24/73 (62.8)
Thomson AJM, 2007	Retro	9/17 (52.9)	8/9 (88.9)	Cai H, 2017	Retro	24/72 (33.3)	13/24 (54.2)
Yasmin H, 2007	Retro	2/19 (10.5)	1/2 (50.0)	Gan L, 2017	RCT	16/80 (20.0)	–

(continued)

Table 14.4 (continued)

Authors	Design	Pregnancy rate	Live birth	Authors	Design	Pregnancy rate	Live birth
Yu D, 2008	Retro	39/85 (45.9)	25/39 (64.1)	Roy KK, 2017	RCT	16/60 (26.7)	9/16 (56.3)
Pabuccu R, 2008	RCT	37/71 (52.1)	22/37 (59.5)	Zhao J, 2017	Pro	63/104 (60.6)	41/63 (65.1)
Robison JK, 2008	Retro	10/15 (66.7)	4/10 (40.0)	Baradwan S, 2018	Retro	22/41 (53.7)	–
Amer MI, 2010	RCT	10/43 (23.3)	–	Hui CYY, 2018	Retro	25/44 (56.8)	19/25 (76.0)
Roy KK, 2010	Retro	36/89 (40.4)	31/89 (34.8)	Xu WZ, 2018	Retro	108/151 (71.5)	80/108 (7401)

Adapted from Guo et al. [10]

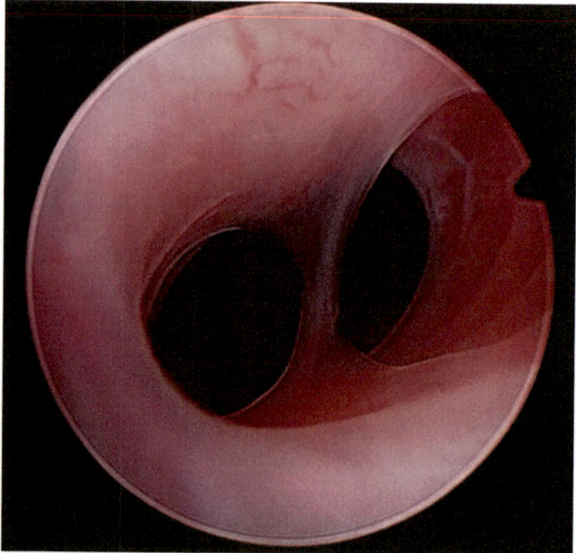

The degree of preoperative adhesions has been well documented to negatively impact postoperative fertility rates. Severe adhesions are more difficult than mild to restore normal uterine anatomy, and often require multiple procedures to achieve restoration of anatomy. Mild, moderate, and severe adhesions have been associated

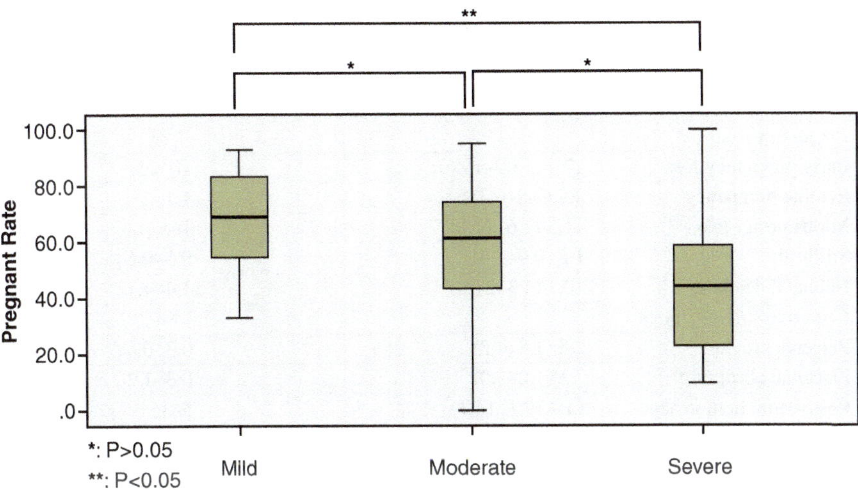

Fig. 14.1 Pregnancy rate after hysteroscopic adhesiolysis. Adapted from Guo et al. [10]

with conception rates of 64.7–69.1%, 53.6–61.3%, and 32.5–44.3%, respectively; see Fig. 14.1 [1, 10]. Two factors are implicated to effect conception when evaluating for the degree of preoperative adhesions: return to normal menstruation, and re-formation of adhesions. Patients with severe adhesions are more likely to have re-formation of IUAs, and are also less likely to have return of normal menstruation compared to patients with moderate or mild IUAs [1].

Hysteroscopic adhesiolysis helps increase both pregnancy and live birth rates, and while this is the goal for a large majority of patients undergoing adhesiolysis, patients need to be counseled on future pregnancy complications. Pregnancies that follow adhesiolysis have been associated with a number of adverse pregnancy complications; see Table 14.5. Compared to the general population, pregnancy after adhesiolysis is associated with increased rates of early pregnancy loss, placental abnormalities, cervical insufficiency, preterm birth, and most significantly complications associated with placenta accreta syndrome. Damage to the endometrium and prior intrauterine surgery increase the risk for development of placenta accreta.

Table 14.5 Prevalence of various adverse pregnancy outcomes for women who conceived after surgical treatment of AS compared with the rates in the general population

Obstetrical complications	IUA population, pooled prevalence (%, 95% CI)	General population (%)
Pregnancy loss		
Early pregnancy loss	17.7 (15.9–19.6)	10–25
Ectopic pregnancy	4.2 (2.8–6.3)	1.1–2
Midtrimester loss	11.5 (7.6–17.8)	1–5
Stillbirth	1.8 (0.9–3.4)	0.5–0.6
Neonatal death	10.3 (4.3–21.8)	1.4–4.1
Obstetrical hemorrhage		
Placenta previa	2.8 (1.8–4.2)	0.3–0.5
Placental abruption	2.3 (1.0–5.0)	0.3–1.2
Postpartum hemorrhage	11.4 (9.1–14.1)	5–15
Others		
Placenta accreta syndrome	10.1 (8.6–11.8)	0.14–0.9
Premature rupture of membrane	5.7 (3.6–8.7)	2–3
Cervical insufficiency	12.5 (3.3–33.5)	1–2
Intrauterine growth restriction	8.4 (6.0–11.6)	8
Preterm birth	14.5 (12.7–16.5)	5–18

Adapted from Guo et al. [10]

14.2 Conclusion

Hysteroscopic adhesiolysis for patients with IUAs has been proven to be a safe and effective surgical intervention. Intraoperative complications are rare, and restoration of a normal uterine cavity is achieved in most cases. Patients with severe IUAs have increased risk of intraoperative complications and are more likely to require more than one procedure to restore normal intrauterine anatomy. Re-formation of IUAs is the most common postoperative complication and is seen in 1/3 of those with severe disease. Adhesiolysis significantly improves conception rates, and most patients are able to conceive within 2 years. Severity of IUA disease is negatively correlated with conception rates, likely due to increased re-formation of IUAs. Patients treated for IUAs should be counseled on increased risks for subsequent pregnancies, specifically the increased risks for placenta accreta syndrome.

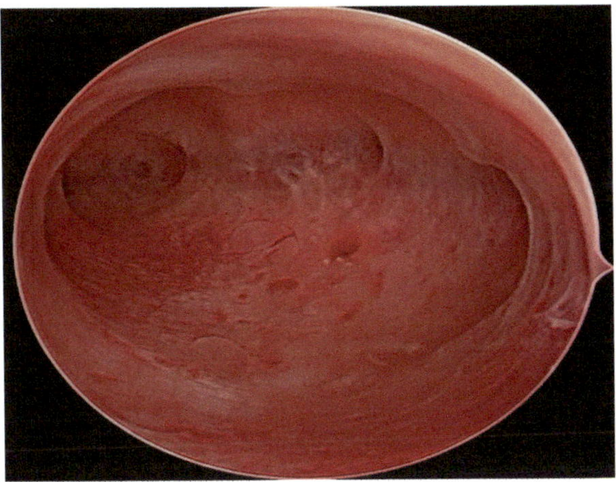

Key Points

1. Hysteroscopic adhesiolysis for patients with IUAs has been proven to be a safe and effective surgical intervention.
2. Intraoperative complications are rare, and restoration of a normal uterine cavity is achieved in most cases.
3. Severe IUAs have increased risk of intraoperative complications and are more likely to require more than one procedure to restore normal intrauterine anatomy.
4. Re-formation of IUAs is the most common postoperative complication and is seen in 1/3 of those with severe disease.
5. Adhesiolysis significantly improves conception rates, and most patients are able to conceive within 2 years.
6. Severity of IUA disease is negatively correlated with conception rates, likely due to increased re-formation of IUAs.
7. IUA-treated women should be counseled about increased risks of obstetric complications including placenta accreta syndrome.

References

1. Yu D, Wong YM, Cheong Y, Xia E, Li TC. Asherman syndrome—one century later. Fertil Steril. 2008;89(4):759–79.
2. Schenker JG, Margalioth EJ. Intrauterine adhesions: an updated appraisal. Fertil Steril. 1982;37(5):593–610.
3. The American Fertility Society. Classifications of adnexal adhesions, distal tubal occlusion, tubal occlusion secondary to tubal ligation, tubal pregnancies, mullerian anomalies and intrauterine adhesions. Fertil Steril. 1988;49(6):944–55.

4. Surgery AEG. AAGL practice report: practice guidelines on intrauterine adhesions developed in collaboration with the European Society of Gynaecological Endoscopy (ESGE). Gynecol Surg. 2017;14(1):6.
5. Sanad AS, Aboulfotouh ME. Hysteroscopic adhesiolysis: efficacy and safety. Arch Gynecol Obstet. 2016;294(2):411–6.
6. Bhandari S, Bhave P, Ganguly I, Baxi A, Agarwal P. Reproductive outcome of patients with Asherman's syndrome: a SAIMS experience. J Reprod Infertil. 2015;16(4):229–35.
7. Hanstede MM, van der Meij E, Goedemans L, Emanuel MH. Results of centralized Asherman surgery, 2003–2013. Fertil Steril. 2015;104(6):1561-8 e1.
8. Khan Z, Goldberg JM. Hysteroscopic management of Asherman's syndrome. J Minim Invasive Gynecol. 2018;25(2):218–28.
9. Malhotra N, Bahadur A, Kalaivani M, Mittal S. Changes in endometrial receptivity in women with Asherman's syndrome undergoing hysteroscopic adhesiolysis. Arch Gynecol Obstet. 2012;286(2):525–30.
10. Guo EJ, Chung JPW, Poon LCY, Li TC. Reproductive outcomes after surgical treatment of Asherman syndrome: a systematic review. Best Pract Res Clin Obstet Gynaecol. 2019;59:98–114.
11. Deans R, Vancaillie T, Ledger W, Liu J, Abbott JA. Live birth rate and obstetric complications following the hysteroscopic management of intrauterine adhesions including Asherman syndrome. Hum Reprod. 2018;33(10):1847–53.
12. Roy KK, Baruah J, Sharma JB, Kumar S, Kachawa G, Singh N. Reproductive outcome following hysteroscopic adhesiolysis in patients with infertility due to Asherman's syndrome. Arch Gynecol Obstet. 2010;281(2):355–61.

Pregnancy and Its Management: Post-Asherman's Treatment

15

Kamal Buckshee and Tanya Buckshee Rohatgi

Diagnostic and therapeutic advances have improved the rates of conception and live births in moderate-to-severe cases of Asherman's syndrome (AS), associated with infertility/subfertility. However, some of these pregnancies may end up into missed abortion/fetal loss/preterm labor/small for dates/intrauterine growth-retarded fetus/cesarean section/cesarean hysterectomy for uncontrolled severe postpartum hemorrhage with abnormal placentation.

The reproductive outcome of these pregnancies depends upon the severity of Asherman's syndrome that was treated and the result achieved. Because of these outcomes, they need regular antenatal checkup, stepwise follow-up, and management.

Critical evaluation before and after conception to delivery and postpartum period is crucial to identify women who are at risk for placental abnormalities, preterm labor, intrauterine growth restriction, and other risk factors for early diagnosis, appropriate, and timely management.

K. Buckshee (✉)
Department of Obstetrics and Gynecology, All India Institute of Medical Science (AIIMS), New Delhi, India

National Academy of Medical Sciences, The Woman Clinic, Noida, India

T. B. Rohatgi
Reproductive Medicine, Reproductive Techniques (IVF), The Woman Clinic, Noida, India

Reproductive Medicine, Reproductive Techniques (IVF), Max Medcentre TM & Max Super Speciality Hospital (Saket), Delhi, India

R. Manchanda (ed.), *Intra Uterine Adhesions*,
https://doi.org/10.1007/978-981-33-4145-6_15

15.1 Important Considerations

- To highlight live birth rate, potential obstetric complications and stepwise management of pregnancies achieved in post-treated cases of Asherman's syndrome (AS).
- To educate and counsel these pregnant women that they are at high risk for severe hemorrhage with abnormal placentation.
- They need to be managed at a tertiary multidisciplinary reproductive care center/hospital.

Refinement and innovations of instruments, hysteroscopic techniques of adhesiolysis, training/retraining, skill development, and awareness of Asherman's syndrome (AS) have revolutionized its diagnosis and management.

Restoration of the uterine cavity with regard to its anatomical size, volume, shape, surface of one or both ostia, regrowth of the denuded endometrium, and improvement in blood flow to the endometrium in moderate-to-severe cases of AS is critical for improving functionality and fertility. However, the inherent risk that led to AS and the trauma caused by surgical procedure/procedures add together and are probably responsible for the adverse outcome [1].

15.2 Conception and Live Birth Rate

Zikopoulos et al. (2004) [2] reported a live delivery rate of 43.5% (20/46) and an overall cumulative live delivery rate was 64.7%. The mean follow-up period was 39.2 ± 4.5 months (Table 15.1).

Roy et al. (2009) [3] reported an overall conception rate of 40.4% following a restructuring of the uterine cavity in cases of infertility (89 patients) due to Asherman's syndrome. The live birth rate was 86.1% and the cumulative pregnancy rate was 97.2% in patients who conceived within 24 months (Table 15.1).

Table 15.1 Conception and live birth rate

	Pregnancy/conception rate					
	(%)	<35 years (%)	>35 years (%)	Natural conception (%)	After IVF/1CSI (%)	Live birth rate (%)
Capella-Allouc et al. (1999) [1]	42.8	62.5	16.6			32.1
Severe AS						
Zikopoulos et al. (2004) [2]				61.9	28.0	43.5
Roy et al. (2009) [3]	40.4					86.1
Chen et al. (2017) [4]	48.2					85.6
Deans et al. (2018) [5]						63.7

Chen et al. (2017) [4] analyzed the data of 332 women treated for Asherman's syndrome. An overall conception rate was 48.2% and the live birth rate was 85.6% (Table 15.1).

Deans et al. (2018) [5] reported 93 births in 79 women following surgery for AS with detailed data being available for 85 births. The live birth rate was 63.7% of the 98 women who achieved pregnancy 21.4% (Table 15.1).

15.3 Obstetric Complications

Zikopoulos et al. (2004) [2] stated that 50.0% of the pregnancies achieved in post-treated cases of Asherman's syndrome ended in premature deliveries after 32 weeks. In one case a planned cesarean hysterectomy was performed for placenta accreta, which was diagnosed antenatally by ultrasound (US), while in the other case perforation of the uterus occurred during manual extraction of placenta accreta.

Roy et al. (2009) [3] reported a miscarriage rate of 11.1%, cesarean section rate of 43.8%, and postpartum hemorrhage (PPH) in 12.5% for the adherent placenta.

Chen et al. (2017) [4] reported a miscarriage rate of 9.4%, postpartum hemorrhage (PPH) 7.9%, adherent placenta 4.3%, and placenta accreta 2.1% (Table 15.3).

Deans et al. (2018) [5] observed abnormal placentation in 17.6%, prematurity in 29.4%, and postpartum hysterectomy in 4.7% (Table 15.3). Most of the studies are retrospective, few are prospective, and the numbers of cases are small.

We need large, multicentric, prospective studies, well planned and structured to understand the etiopathogenesis responsible for the unfavorable reproductive outcome. The obstetric prognosis is to be correlated to the severity of AS, number of surgical procedures, and maternal and neonatal morbidity and mortality (Fig. 15.1).

15.4 Pregnancy: Stepwise Management

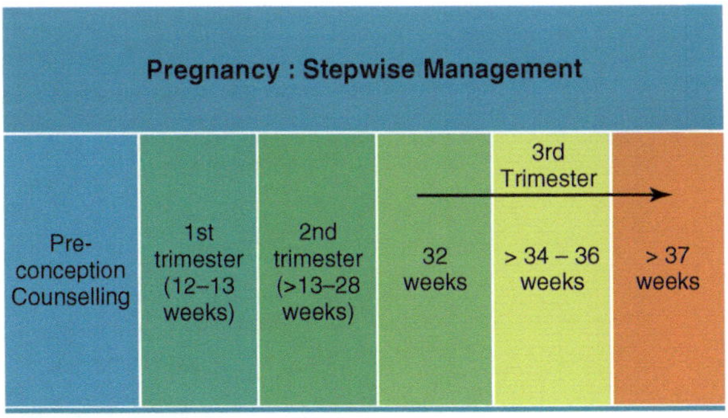

Fig. 15.1 Pregnancy: stepwise management

15.5 Preconception Management: Follow-Up Visit—After 8 Weeks of Index Surgery

- To educate, counsel, and create awareness among couples wanting to conceive about the conception rate, live birth rate, and possible reproductive outcomes of the pregnancies achieved following treatment of Asherman's syndrome.
- They should be informed that live birth rate and obstetric complications will depend upon the severity of Asherman's syndrome that was treated (Figs. 15.2 and 15.3).

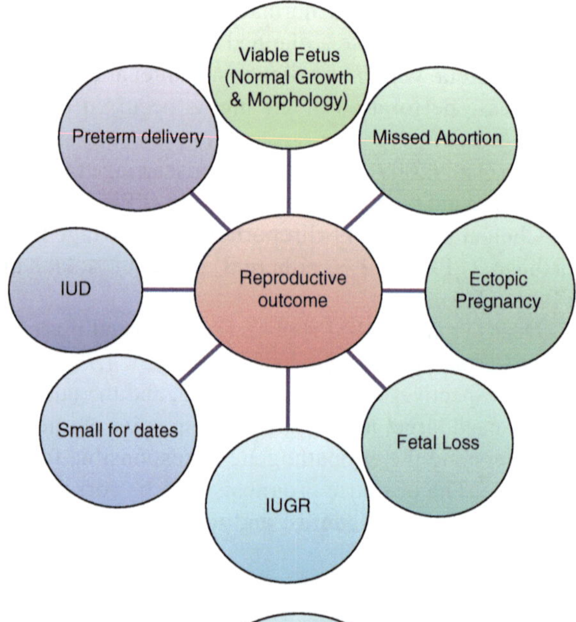

Fig. 15.2 Reproductive profile and treatment outcome (**a**)

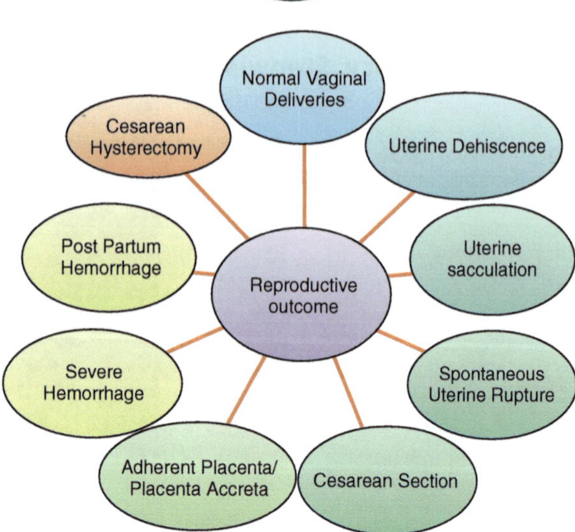

Fig. 15.3 Reproductive profile and treatment outcome (**b**)

- Advantages of regular antenatal checkups and follow-up of stepwise management.
- A detailed history (cesarean section, intrauterine surgery, menstrual, obstetric, surgical, and other history), clinical evaluation of the patient, review of preoperative and postoperative hysteroscopic findings to assess the severity/degree of Asherman's syndrome before surgery and after surgery from the results achieved.
- Restoration of the uterine cavity with regard to size, volume and shape, endometrial lining, regular/irregular and vascular flow to the endometrium.
- To know if there is a need for relook hysteroscopic surgery, pelvic ultrasound (US), transabdominal (TA), and transvaginal (TVS) are to be performed with color flow, 3D, and evaluation of the cervical canal on days 17–18 of the menstrual cycle.
- Assess the fertility status of the couple. Consent for planning pregnancy to be taken after the patient and her partner are informed and explained about the possible reproductive outcome after the index surgery.
- Record the data systematically and inform the patient to visit the treating obstetrician once the pregnancy test is positive along with the relevant blood tests and pelvic ultrasound (US) at 8–10 weeks of pregnancy.

15.6 Pregnancy and Its Management: Maternal and Fetal Surveillance

- **First trimester** (*8–10 weeks*): A detailed history, clinical evaluation, and review of blood tests. A transabdominal pelvic (TA) and TV ultrasound to detect fetal viability, or missed abortion or ectopic pregnancy. If the fetus is viable, repeat ultrasound at 12–13 weeks of pregnancy.
  Level I ultrasound (*12–13 weeks*): Assess if the fetus is viable or there is missed abortion. If viable, assess growth, morphology, placental implantation, blood flow, cervical length, and biochemical screening for risk assessment of trisomies (first-trimester screening).
- **Second trimester**: Anomaly scans at 18–19 weeks' pregnancy to include placental localization, risk assessment for preterm labor or delivery, and assessment of fetal growth and morphology [6].
  After performing the anomaly scan, identify women at risk for placenta previa or low-lying placenta or placenta accreta. If the placenta is low lying (less than 20 mm from the internal os) or previa (covering the os), then a follow-up scan should be done by a skilled ultrasonologist at 32 weeks of gestation [7].
  Since prematurity is one of the potential risks in post-Asherman-treated pregnancies identify asymptomatic women at risk of preterm labor.
  A history of spontaneous preterm birth (up to 34 + 0 weeks of pregnancy) or midtrimester loss (from 16 + 0 weeks of pregnancy onwards) or transvaginal ultrasound scan between 16 + 0 weeks and 24 + 0 weeks of pregnancy indicates shortening of the cervix (less than 25 mm); hence consider prophylactic

cervical cerclage. If there is a widening of the endocervical canal or bulging of membranes in the cervical canal then think of rescue cervical cerclage. Since these women are at increased risk of preterm labor, discuss with the patient and her partner the advantages and disadvantages of the procedure. If the clinical assessment and ultrasound suggest that the pregnant woman is suspected of preterm labor at 29 + 6 weeks' pregnancy or less, treatment for preterm labor has to be started. If transvaginal ultrasound measurement of cervical length is less than 15 mm, it indicates a likelihood of birth within 48 h [8]. Offer antenatal corticosteroids to women between 24 + 0 and 33 + 6 weeks of pregnancy, who are suspected of, diagnosed with, or in established preterm labor.
Magnesium sulfate is given for neuroprotection for women between 24 + 0 and 29 + 6 weeks of pregnancy who are in established preterm labor or having a planned preterm birth within 24 h [8].

15.6.1 Diagnosis of Fetal Growth Restriction (FGR) or Small-for-Gestational-Age (SGA) Fetus

Fetal abdominal circumference (AC) or estimated fetal weight (EFW) <10th centile for the period of gestation can be used to diagnose SGA fetus. A low level of PAPP-A (<0.415 MoM), the first-trimester marker, can also be considered a risk factor for the delivery of a SGA neonate. Doppler flow at 20–24 weeks of pregnancy has a moderate predictive value for a severe SGA neonate [6].

Women with SGA fetus between 24 + 0 and 35 + 6 weeks of gestation, where delivery is being considered, should receive a single course of antenatal corticosteroids. Magnesium sulfate is administered for neuroprotection in women going to deliver before 30 weeks of gestation [8].

- **Third trimester (28–32 weeks)**: Assess fetal growth, risk of preterm delivery, and abnormal placentation. In asymptomatic women with a persistent low-lying placenta or placenta previa at 32 weeks of gestation, an additional TVS is recommended at around 36 weeks of gestation to inform and discuss the mode of delivery with the couple and their family members. Cervical length measurement is useful in deciding the mode of delivery. A short cervical length on TVS before 34 weeks of gestation increases the risk of preterm emergency delivery and massive hemorrhage at cesarean section. These women should attend the hospital immediately if they experience any bleeding, including spotting, contractions, or pain (including vague suprapubic period-like aches). Asymptomatic women with placenta previa confirmed at the 32-week follow-up scan and managed at home should have help and transport available 24 × 7 to help them and to shift them to the hospital immediately when required [7].
  32–36 weeks: A single course of antenatal corticosteroid therapy is recommended between 34 + 0 and 35 + 6 weeks of gestation for pregnant women with a low-lying placenta or placenta previa preferably before 34 weeks of

gestation in women at higher risk of preterm birth. Late preterm (34 + 0 to 36 + 6 weeks of gestation) delivery should be considered for women presenting with placenta previa or a low-lying placenta and a history of vaginal bleeding or other associated risk factors for preterm delivery.

Before delivery, all women with antenatal diagnosis of placenta previa or abnormal placentation should have a discussion along with their partners regarding delivery, indications for blood transfusion, and cesarean hysterectomy [7].

Consider vertical skin and/or uterine incisions when the fetus is in a transverse lie to avoid the placenta, particularly below 28 weeks of gestation. If the placenta is transected during the uterine incision, immediately clamp the umbilical cord after the delivery of the fetus to avoid excessive fetal blood loss.

If pharmacological measures fail to control hemorrhage, initiate intrauterine tamponade and/or surgical hemostatic techniques sooner rather than later. Early recourse to hysterectomy is recommended if conservative medical and surgical interventions prove ineffective. Previous cesarean delivery and presence of an anterior low-lying placenta or placenta previa should alert the obstetrician of the higher risk of placenta accreta.

Ultrasound imaging is highly accurate when performed by a skilled operator with experience in diagnosing placenta accreta. Non-contrast magnetic resonance imaging (MRI) may be used to complement ultrasound imaging to assess the depth of invasion and lateral extension of myometrial invasion, especially with posterior placentation and/or in women with ultrasound signs suggesting parametrial invasion. Women diagnosed with placenta accreta should be cared for by a multidisciplinary team in a tertiary reproductive care center/hospital with expertise in diagnosing and managing invasive placentation [7].

In the absence of risk factors for preterm delivery in women with placenta accreta, planned delivery at 35 + 0 to 36 + 6 weeks of gestation provides the best balance between fetal maturity and risk of unscheduled delivery [7].

The elective delivery of women with placenta accreta should be managed by a multidisciplinary team (senior anesthetists, obstetricians, gynecologists, vascular/oncology surgeon/intervention radiologist). There is limited evidence to support uterus-preserving surgery in placenta percreta.

These women should be informed of the high risk of peripartum and secondary complications, including the need for secondary hysterectomy. If at the time of an elective repeat cesarean section, where both mother and baby are stable, it is apparent that placenta percreta is present on opening the abdomen, the cesarean section should be delayed until the appropriate staff and resources have assembled and adequate blood products are available. This may involve closure of the maternal abdomen and an urgent transfer to a specialist unit for delivery. In case of unsuspected placenta accreta diagnosed after the birth of the baby, the placenta should be left in situ and an emergency hysterectomy should be performed; patient and her family members should be made aware that placental pathology is associated with high morbidity and risk of maternal death, despite advances in ultrasonography, well-established surgical treatment, and multidisciplinary medical care [7].

15.7 Evidences

Live birth in patients treated for moderate-to-severe Asherman's syndrome with infertility/subfertility is an important milestone. Zikopoulos et al. (2004) [2] reviewed ten studies of women with Asherman's syndrome treated by various adhesiolysis methods. They stated that probably about 40.0% of patients can be expected to deliver following the index surgery. In their study, live delivery rate following adhesiolysis was 43.5% (20/46) [2]. However, following natural conception it was 61.9% vs. 28.0% in patients treated by IVF/ICSI (Table 15.1).

Case report series of patients treated for severe AS pregnancy rate was 42.8% and live birth rate was 32.1% [1]. These rates were higher (62.5%) in younger women <35 years vs. 16.6% in women >35 years (61.9%). The results are encouraging. However, many studies fail to present their data according to the severity of Asherman's syndrome. The conception/live birth rates in treated cases of AS are higher in mild cases as compared to those in moderate and severe. They vary from 21.0% to 60.7% in mild, 30.0% to 53.4% in moderate, and 25.0% to 46.7% in severe cases (Table 15.2).

It is difficult to compare conception/live delivery rates due to lack of uniform classification, different techniques used for adhesiolysis, retrospective or prospective study, age of the patients, type of population, severity/grade of AS treated, anatomical restructuring, and functionality of the uterine cavity achieved after adhesiolysis and other variables. Zikopoulos et al. (2004) [2] observed a very high rate of preterm delivery (50.0%) after 32 weeks' pregnancy. Planned cesarean hysterectomy was performed for placenta accreta in one case, which was diagnosed antenatally by ultrasound (US), while in the other case perforation of the uterus occurred during manual extraction of placenta accreta. Cesarean hysterectomy was performed in two cases, due to placenta accreta. Placenta accreta was the most common life-threatening complication observed in pregnancies achieved following adhesiolysis. Its incidence was 8.0%. The probable reason for abnormal placentation being defective is lamina basal possibly occurring after adhesiolysis [2].

Capella-Allouc et al. (1999) [1] stated that normal size and shape of uterine cavity are essential to carry a pregnancy to term. Capella-Allouc et al. (1999) [1] reported 15 pregnancies in 12 patients of severe Asherman's syndrome (SAS) after repeated surgical procedures. The pregnancy rate after treatment was 42.8% (12/28) and the live birth rate was 32.1% (9/28). The outcome of these

Table 15.2 Severity of Asherman's syndrome and subsequent fertility

Zikopoulos et al (2004) [2]	33.3%	44.4%	46.7%	Live delivery rate
	Mild	**Moderate**	**Severe**	
Roy et al. (2009) [3]	58.0%	30.0%	33.3%	Conception rate
Chen et al. (2017) [4]	60.7%	53.4%	25.0%	
	Grade I	**Grade II**	**Grade III**	**Grade IV**
Deans et al. (2018) [5]	21.4%	36.7%	27.6%	13.3%

Table 15.3 Reproductive outcome in treated AS pregnancies

	Premature deliveries (%)	Miscarriage (%)	CS (%)	PPH (%)	Adherent placenta (%)	Placenta accreta (%)	Abnormal placentation (%)
Zikopoulos et al. (2004) [2]	50.0				8		
Roy et al. (2009) [3]		11.1	43.8	12.5			
Chen et al. (2017) [4]		9.4		7.9	4.3	2.1	
Deans et al (2018) [5]	29.4			4.7			17.6

pregnancies was two first-trimester missed abortions, three second-trimester fetal losses, one second-trimester termination of pregnancy for multiple fetal abnormalities, and nine live births in nine different patients. In patients less than 35 years of age, 10 out of 16 conceived (62.5%) versus 2 out of 12 (16.6%) who were >35 years. In nine patients with live births, one cesarean hysterectomy (3.57%) was performed for placenta accreta and ligation of hypogastric arteries was done in one case for severe hemorrhage (3.5%) and placenta accreta (7%). Reconstruction of a functional uterine cavity resulted in 42.8% pregnancy rate (Table 15.1). Their study highlights that almost 50.0% of patients conceived and almost one-third had live births. Severe obstetric complications reported in subsequent pregnancies following treatment of AS were spontaneous uterine rupture occurring during pregnancy, the cause being fundal perforation during surgical treatment of AS, uterine sacculation, uterine dehiscence, and placenta accreta. Incidence of placenta accreta reported varied from 9.0% to 22.2% [1]. In spite of high chance of pregnancy and live births following treatment, these pregnancies are frequently complicated by premature births and abnormal placenta-related morbidity for the mother and the offspring (Table 15.3).

Reported rate of miscarriage varies from 9.0% to 11%, postpartum hemorrhage (PPH) 4.7–12.5%, and abnormal placentation 17.6%. The reported rate of cesarean section is very high. It varies from 43.8% to 69.0% (Tables 15.3 and 15.5). Bhandari et al. (2015) [9] conducted a prospective study on 60 patients with AS. They observed that pregnancy rate correlated significantly with the severity of adhesions and postoperative endometrial echo pattern. Sixteen women conceived with three missed abortions, eleven live births, three preterm, one preterm neonate died due to respiratory distress syndrome, two ongoing, and one had PPH, due to retained placenta (Table 15.4).

Malhotra et al. (2012) [10] analyzed endometrial thickness and Doppler flow in patients with Asherman's syndrome and found that although there was an improvement in endometrial thickness, the vascularity did not improve indicating that endometrial functionality was not achieved. Thus, surgery restructures the distorted anatomy and probably improves endometrial growth and thickness but

Table 15.4 Reproductive profile according to severity and treatment outcome [7]

Total		Pregnancy	Miscarriage	Preterm	Live birth	Ongoing
Mild	13	7 (53.8)	1 (7.7)	1 (7.7)	5 (38.5)	1 (7.7)
Moderate	26	7 (26.5)	2 (7.7)	0 (0.0)	4 (15.4)	1 (3.8)
Severe	21	2 (9.5)	0 (0.0)	1 (4.8)	1 (4.8)	0 (0.0)

Table 15.5 Obstetric outcomes from live births with complete datasets in women [5]

	First live birth of total, *n* (% of total births)	Second live birth following surgery, *n* (% of total births)	Third live birth following surgery, *n* (% of total births)	Overall, following surgery, *n* (% births)
Number of births	71[a] (83.5)	13 (15.3)	1 (1.2)	85 (100)
Cesarean delivery[b]	**49 (69.0)**	**8 (61.5)**	**1 (100)**	**58 (68.2)**
Antepartum bleeding[b]	2 (2.4)	0 (0)	0 (0)	2 (2.4)
Placenta previa[b]	**6 (8.5)**	**1 (7.7)**	**0 (0)**	**7 (8.2)**
Placenta accreta[b]	**6 (8.5)**	**0 (0)**	**1 (100)**	**7 (8.2)**
Vasa previa[b]	1 (1.4)	0 (0)	0 (0)	1 (1.2)
Manual removal of placenta[b]	**12 (16.9)**	**1 (7.7)**	**0 (0)**	**13 (15.3)**
Postpartum hemorrhage[b]	**12 (16.9)**	**1 (7.7)**	**0 (0)**	**13 (15.3)**
Blood transfusion[b]	3 (4.2)	1 (7.7)	0 (0)	4 (4.7)
Prolonged postpartum bleeding >6 weeks[b]	1 (1.4)	0 (0)	0 (0)	1 (1.2)
Postpartum hysterectomy[b]	**3 (4.2)**	**1 (7.7)**	**0 (0)**	**4 (4.7)**

[a]Obstetric outcomes were only available for 71/79 women who achieved live birth
[b]Denotes the number of events as a proportion of first, second, or third live births following index surgery

does not restore functionality of the endometrium. Reduced blood flow in subendometrial zone has been observed even when endometrial thickness appeared normal [11]. Bhandari et al.'s (2015) [9] study highlights that endometrial lining and echo pattern improved significantly after adhesiolysis. In their study no case of placenta accreta was observed, with limitation of the study being small number of cases. Deans et al. (2018) [5] conducted a retrospective and recall basis study. Out of 124 patients 98 conceived, 29 had miscarriage, and 79 had live births. Their result indicates an increase in the risk of placenta accreta. Yu et al. (2008) [12], March et al. (2011) [13], and Deans et al. (2018) [5] suggest a trebling of this rate to 8%. Premature births and low birth weight were common events (Table 15.5).

Their study indicated that chance of pregnancy was 79.0%, live birth 63.7%, miscarriage 23.4%, abnormal placentation 17.6%, postpartum hysterectomy 4.7%, and prematurity 29.4%. Their pregnancy rates were higher, but obstetric

Table 15.6 Neonatal outcomes with complete datasets [5]

	First live birth following surgery	Second live birth following surgery	Third live birth following surgery	Overall
Number of babies, *n* (% of total babies)	72[a] (83.7)	13 (15.1)	1 (1.2)	86 (100)
Mean weight, *n* in kg (range)	3.08 (0.9–4.35)	3.13 (2–3.85)	3.32[c]	3.08 (0.9–4.35)
Preterm pre-labor rupture of membranes[b], *n* (%)	1 (1.4)	0 (0)	0 (0)	1 (1.2)
Preterm birth <37 weeks' gestation[b], *n* (%)	23 (31.9)	2 (15.4)	0 (0)	25 (29.1)
Preterm birth <30 weeks' gestation[b], *n* (%)	3 (4.2)	0 (0)	0 (0)	3 (3.5)
Mean gestation of premature birth weeks, *n* (range)	31 (20–36)	34[c]	–	31 (20–36)
Neonatal deaths[b], *n* (%)	1 (1.4)	1 (7.7)	0 (0)	2 (2.4)

[a]72 Neonatal outcomes are reported as one woman had a twin pregnancy
[b]Denotes the number of events as a proportion of first, second, or third births following index surgery
[c]No range given as only one delivery

and neonatal complications also increased. They are of the view that there is an altered biochemical or vascular environment, which is responsible for impaired implantation, which in turn results in poorer obstetric and neonatal outcome (Table 15.6).

One might face a very challenging situation while managing pregnancies achieved in treated cases of AS by coming across an asymptomatic patient having regular antenatal checkup and ultrasonography with no abnormal findings detected and observing abnormal placentation during cesarean section. Engelbrechtsen et al. (2015) [14] reported a case of adherent placenta due to Asherman's syndrome, which was not detected in a patient who was thoroughly examined with sonography during pregnancy. Two-dimensional ultrasonography has a sensitivity of 77–90.7%, a specificity of 96–98%, a positive predictive value of 65–93%, and a negative predictive value of 98% for detecting placenta accreta. Magnetic resonance imaging (MRI) has a sensitivity of 80–85% and specificity of 65–100%. Use of MRI in conjunction with 2D ultrasonography especially when the placenta is located posterior and history of previous cesarean section/suspicion would be helpful. In women with antenatal diagnosis of adherent placenta/placenta accreta, the obstetrician along with her multidisciplinary team should be prepared to handle the situation. In these cases there is reduced blood loss and need for blood transfusion is also less. This case highlights that a skilled ultrasonologist familiar with reproductive outcome should scan pregnancies achieved post-Asherman's treatment. If there is suspicion, the patient should have a planned cesarean section with a skilled senior obstetrician, along with skilled anesthetist, intervention radiologist/vascular surgeon, and blood bank and donors who should be informed in advance due to the risk of severe hemorrhage. The reported incidence of placenta accreta is 13–14% with previous Asherman's syndrome [14]. Patients treated for moderate-to-severe AS should be closely monitored for early diagnosis of spontaneous rupture of uterus and placental implantation abnormalities in order to decrease maternal fetal and neonatal morbidity and mortality.

Large, multicenter collaborative, prospective, well-structured, clinical, and research studies are needed to evaluate the obstetric complications and fetal and neonatal outcome in pregnancies achieved following treatment. These outcomes are to be correlated with the severity of AS, number of surgeries performed, extent of anatomical size, and shape and functionality of uterine cavity restored. Angiogenesis in relation to the endometrium, myometrium, and cervical competency should be assessed along with a long-term follow-up of 5 years of fetal and neonatal outcome. Hysteroscopic centers of excellence are needed where a multidisciplinary skilled team (surgeon, anesthetist, imaging technology, skilled radiologist, staff, and instruments) is available in managing moderate-to-severe cases of AS along with standard protocol/guidelines at a tertiary reproductive center where facilities exist to manage high-risk pregnancies achieved after treatment of Asherman's syndrome.

15.8 Management

1. Individualize management of pregnancies achieved after treatment of Asherman's syndrome from preconception to delivery and postpartum period.
2. Systematic stepwise management from conception to delivery and postpartum period is crucial for early diagnosis and appropriate and timely management of potential risks/complications to reduce fetal, neonatal, and maternal morbidity and mortality.
3. In view of the risk of severe life-threatening hemorrhage in cases of abnormal placentation, these pregnant women need awareness/preparedness/consent for admission at a tertiary multidisciplinary hospital for blood transfusion and cesarean section/cesarean hysterectomy.
4. Educate, counsel, and promote awareness among physicians, gynecologists, ultrasonologist/radiologists, anesthetists, surgeons, and nurses that pregnancies occurring after treatment of Asherman's syndrome are at high risk for life-threatening obstetric complications.
5. Since these pregnancies are prone to abnormal placentation with a risk of severe hemorrhage and even maternal death, these cases should be managed at a tertiary care reproductive center/hospital.
6. Audit conception rate/live birth rate, obstetric complications, and cesarean section rate/cesarean hysterectomy fetal and neonatal outcome.

Key Points

1. Live birth/delivery rates and a real chance of motherhood/parenthood have increased following treatment of Asherman's syndrome.
2. Pregnancies achieved following treatment of moderate-to-severe Asherman's syndrome should be considered as high-risk obstetric cases.
3. These pregnancies are prone to missed abortion, fetal loss, preterm delivery, intrauterine growth restriction, premature placenta previa, abnormal placentation, with severe postpartum hemorrhage, cesarean section, and cesarean hysterectomy. Prematurity and placenta accreta are the common complications.
4. Educate, counsel, and create awareness of potential risks/complications associated with pregnancies achieved post-Asherman's treatment.
5. Antenatal diagnosis of abnormal placentation/placenta accreta spectrum using ultrasound aids, early diagnosis, planning time, and mode of delivery, thereby reducing blood loss and fetal, neonatal, and maternal morbidity and mortality.
6. Placenta accreta is the most common life-threatening complication observed in pregnancies achieved following adhesiolysis.
7. These pregnancies should be managed by senior, experienced, skilled team of an obstetrician, oncologist/vascular surgeon, intervention radiologist, anesthetist, staff, and blood bank at a multidisciplinary tertiary reproductive care/center/hospital.
8. History of previous cesarean delivery with the presence of anterior low-lying placenta or placenta previa in the current pregnancy should alert the obstetrician of the high risk of placenta accreta.

References

1. Capella-Allouc S, Morsad F, Rongières-Bertrand C, Taylor S, Fernandez H. Hysteroscopic treatment of severe Asherman's syndrome and subsequent fertility. Hum Reprod. 1999;14(5):1230–3.
2. Zikopoulos KA, Kolibianakis EM, Platteau P, et al. Live delivery rates in subfertile women with Asherman's syndrome after hysteroscopic adhesiolysis using the resectoscope or the Versa point system. Reprod BioMed Online. 2004;8:720.
3. Roy KK, Baruah J, Sharma JB, Kumar S, Kachawa G, Singh N. Reproductive outcome following hysteroscopic adhesiolysis in patients with infertility due to Asherman's syndrome. Arch Gynecol Obstet. 2010;281(2):355–61.
4. Chen L, Zhang H, Wang Q, Xie F, Gao S, Song Y, Dong J, Feng H, Xie K, Sui L. Reproductive outcomes in patients with intrauterine adhesions following hysteroscopic adhesiolysis: experience from the largest Women's Hospital in China. J Minim Invasive Gynecol. 2017;24(2):299–304. https://doi.org/10.1016/j.jmig.2016.10.018.
5. Deans R, Vancaillie T, Ledger W, Liu J, Abbott JA. Live birth rate and obstetric complications following the hysteroscopic management of intrauterine adhesions including Asherman syndrome. Hum Reprod. 2018;33(10):1847–53. https://doi.org/10.1093/humrep/dey237.
6. Royal College of Obstetricians and Gynecologists. The investigation and management of the small-for-gestational-age fetus. Green-top guideline no. 31. 2013. 2nd ed. https://www.rcog.org.uk/globalassets/documents/guidelines/gtg_31.pdf. Accessed 10 Sep 2017.

7. Jauniaux E, Alfirevic Z, Bhide AG, Belfort MA, Burton GJ, Collins SL, Dornan S, Jurkovic D, Kayem G, Kingdom J, Silver R, Sentilhes L. Placenta praevia and placenta accreta: diagnosis and management: green-top guideline No. 27a. BJOG. 2019;126(1):e1–e48.
8. Preterm labour and birth NICE guideline [NG25] Published date: November 2015 https://www.nice.org.uk/guidance/ng25?unlid=9291036072016213201257.
9. Bhandari S, Bhave P, Ganguly I, Baxi A, Agarwal P. Reproductive outcome of patients with Asherman's syndrome: a SAIMS experience. J Reprod Infertil. 2015;16(4):229–35.
10. Malhotra N, Bahadur A, Kalaivani M, Mittal S. Changes in endometrial receptivity in women with Asherman's syndrome undergoing hysteroscopic adhesiolysis. Arch Gynecol Obstet. 2012;286(2):525–30.
11. Zhao J, Zhang Q, Li Y. The effect of endometrial thickness and pattern measured by ultrasonography on pregnancy outcomes during IVF-ET cycles. Reprod Biol Endocrinol. 2012;10:100.
12. Yu D, Wong YM, Cheong Y, Xia E, Li TC. Asherman syndrome—one century later. Fertil Steril. 2008;89:759–79.
13. March CM. Management of Asherman's syndrome. Reprod BioMed Online. 2011;23:63–76.
14. Engelbrechtsen L, Langhoff-Roos J, JoergenKjer J, Istre O. Placenta accreta: adherent placenta due to Asherman syndrome. Clin Case Rep. 2015;3(3):175–8. https://doi.org/10.1002/ccr3.194.

Placental Complications Associated with Asherman's Syndrome

16

Salvatore Giovanni Vitale, Federica Di Guardo, and Antonio Simone Laganà

The Asherman's syndrome occurs mainly as a result of trauma to the gravid uterine cavity determining its partial or complete obliteration with the possibility of cervical canal involvement [1–4]. The development of intrauterine adhesions is associated, in approximately 90% of cases, with intrauterine curettage after pregnancy; therefore, emptying of the uterine cavity after abortion or delivery should be performed gently and preferable under ultrasonic guidance or by hysteroscopy [5].

However, Asherman's syndrome can also occur in a nongravid uterus as a result of procedures damaging the endometrium [6]. Despite the widespread use of minimally invasive techniques such as office hysteroscopy for treatment of intrauterine affections, Asherman's syndrome represents one of the main long-term complications associated also with interventions having a minimal impact on the uterine cavity [7]. Moreover, it is well documented that multiple uterine interventions are more likely to cause intrauterine adhesions than a single operation [6]. Hysteroscopy and office hysteroscopy represent the gold standard both for diagnosis and treatment of Asherman's syndrome. Nowadays hysteroscopic adhesiolysis is considered an effective treatment of intrauterine adhesions, with an overall conception rate of 40% following the procedure [8]. However, although the hysteroscopic surgery has reached significant advancing during the last 10 years, the treatment of mild-to-severe Asherman's syndrome still represents a challenge. Consequences of endometrium dysfunction and uterine cavity trauma result in conditions such as menstrual abnormalities, dysmenorrhea, and infertility [4].

S. G. Vitale (✉) · F. Di Guardo
Obstetrics and Gynecology Unit, Department of General Surgery and Medical Surgical Specialties, University of Catania, Catania, Italy
e-mail: sgvitale@unict.it

A. S. Laganà
Department of Obstetrics and Gynecology, "Filippo Del Ponte" Hospital, University of Insubria, Varese, Italy

R. Manchanda (ed.), *Intra Uterine Adhesions*,
https://doi.org/10.1007/978-981-33-4145-6_16

Considering conceiving after Asherman's syndrome treatments, Yu et al. [9] demonstrated in a recent study of 85 cases with 109 surgical interventions that women who remained amenorrheic had a significantly lower chance of conception (18.2% versus 50%). In line with this data, the conception rate for women with regular cavity at second-look hysteroscopy was 59.1% versus 11.8% for those who showed reformation of adhesions.

Nevertheless, when the pregnancy occurs in women with a history of Asherman's syndrome, there is a high risk of severe complications such as spontaneous abortion, recurrent pregnancy loss, preterm delivery, intrauterine growth restriction, uterine rupture, and even placenta previa or accretism [2–10].

In pregnant women, the trauma of endometrium may lead to alterations of the decidual layers, especially the one that separates the decidua basalis from the placental villi, also known as Nitabuch's layer. Raissa Nitabuch was the first who described this fibrinous layer in the decidua as the area where the placenta detaches from the uterine wall after delivery. The decidual fibrin layer was just an accidental finding in her study, mainly focused on describing the anatomical connection between the intervillous space and the maternal vasculature. What is known about the function of the Nitabuch's layer is that it plays a crucial role in the prevention of excessively deep implantation [11]. The marked increasing of abnormal implantation incidence, especially in developing countries, is probably attributable to the increased frequency and number of operative procedures disturbing the integrity of the decidua's basalis [12]. In this regard, several studies investigating specimens following termination of pregnancy or curettage procedure demonstrated the presence of myometrial fibers in a large quantity of the cases, thus clearly raising the issue of considering the endometrial injury like a precursor to abnormal placental invasion. Consistent with the elements highlighted above, cases of invasive placentation in patients with Asherman's syndrome may refer to endometrial trauma leading to defects or absence of decidua basalis with incomplete development of Nitabuch's layer [13].

16.1 Placenta Accreta

Placenta accreta develops when the anchoring villi of the placenta adhere directly to the surface of the myometrium without intervening decidua [14, 15]. Placenta accreta is described as an abnormal placentation leading to pregnancy complications, possibly resulting in obstetric hemorrhage, disseminated intravascular coagulation, and, in the worst scenarios, uterine rupture or even death [16]. Therefore, placenta accreta has today become the leading reason for cesarean hysterectomy in several centers [17, 18].

Asherman's patients achieving pregnancy reported high significant risk of obstetric complications including placenta accreta [19, 20]. Although several studies evaluated obstetric outcomes in pregnant women with previous Asherman's syndrome, few and sparse data are reported. Literature background has showed a number of cases about this element, but no large observational studies are available so far.

The incidence of placenta accreta in patients with previous Asherman's syndrome was estimated to be 13–14% by Schenker and Margalioth in 1982 [2]. On the other hand, Roy et al. [8] found an incidence of postpartum hemorrhage due to placenta accreta in 12.5% of the 89 women who had undergone hysteroscopic adhesiolysis due to Asherman's syndrome. Fernandez et al. [21] reported an incidence of placenta accreta in patients with previous treatments for severe Asherman's syndrome: specifically, they reported that 3 (14.3%) patients of 21 had either hysterectomy or hypogastric artery ligation for placenta accreta. This does not match with the findings of Miller et al. [22], reporting a placenta accreta rate of 1 on 2500 deliveries in a study observation from 1985 to 1994. Moreover, a review of cases from 1982 found an incidence of 1 in 533 deliveries [23].

Although thc last two studies showed cesarean deliveries and maternal age as main risk factors for placenta accreta, there was no mention of previous treatment for Asherman's syndrome.

Nevertheless, a placenta accreta incidence of 3 on 21 patients represents an increase in this serious obstetric complication. Yu et al. [9] in a recent study of 85 cases with 109 operative procedures found that women who remained in amenorrhea had a significantly lower chance of conception (18.2% versus 50%). Similarly, the conception rate for women with a regular cavity at second-look hysteroscopy was 59.1% versus 11.8% for those who still showed adhesions. To date, two-dimensional ultrasonography represents the best method to detect placenta accreta with a sensitivity of 77–90.7%, a specificity of 96–98%, a positive predictive value of 65–93%, and a negative predictive value of 98% [24, 25]. Magnetic resonance imaging (MRI) may also be helpful to confirm the diagnosis, since it has a sensitivity of 80–85% and a specificity of 65–100% [26]. MRI should be performed in association with the conventional ultrasonography [27], especially when the placenta is difficult to be detected, being located on the posterior uterine wall. However, it is important to mention that MRI does not represent a good prognostic tool to change the surgical management in cases of placenta accreta [28]. Several retrospective studies have shown that women with an antenatal diagnosis of placenta accreta reported less quantity of blood loss and less necessity to undergo blood transfusion than women in whom the abnormal placentation was diagnosed during the cesarean section [29, 30]. Good clinical practice advices to examine patients with a previous history of intrauterine surgery or Asherman's syndrome by a skilled sonographer for possibility of abnormal placentation. In case of abnormal placentation suspicion, the patient should be scheduled for elective cesarean section performed by skilled clinician's due to risk of severe postpartum hemorrhage [31].

16.2 Placenta Previa

Placenta previa is defined as the presence of placental tissue extending over the internal cervical orifice. Placenta previa sequelae may include severe bleeding and preterm birth, as well as the need for cesarean delivery. It seems that the defective uterine endometrium as well as the obliterated uterine cavity may predispose to placenta previa due to the decidual deficiency typical of Asherman's syndrome. Moreover, the presence of intrauterine adhesions or previous interventions on the uterine cavity can lead to a placental defective implantation even covering the cervix.

Consistent with these elements, several studies showed placenta previa reported as obstetrics outcomes of intrauterine adhesions. A recent study reported that complications of delivery including placenta previa were significantly higher in patients with a history of Asherman's syndrome compared with controls [32]. This result had been already noted by Feng et al. [33], reporting placenta previa as one of the obstetric outcomes in women with a history of intrauterine adhesions.

Diagnosis of placenta previa is commonly on sonographic identification of echogenic homogeneous placenta extending over the internal cervical os during the second- or third-trimester ultrasound scan. The distance (millimeters) between the internal cervical os and the inferior edge of the placenta should be described in the diagnostic report [34]. To date, vaginal examination should be avoided and is not needed given the superiority of ultrasound diagnosis. Transabdominal ultrasonography represents the first sonographic approach in most pregnant women. An additional transvaginal ultrasound scan may be performed when optimal visualization of the relationship between the placenta and cervix is needed. If the distance between the edge of the placenta and the cervical os is ≤2 cm on transabdominal ultrasound, transvaginal sonography may be required to better define placental position and make the diagnosis. However, when available, three-dimensional ultrasound scan may improve accuracy over transvaginal sonography [35]. Translabial (transperineal) ultrasound imaging is considered an alternative technique to transvaginal ultrasound providing optimal images of the cervix and placenta [36]. Finally, MRI is commonly not used for diagnosis of placenta previa because of its high cost, limited availability, and well-established safety and accuracy of transvaginal sonography [34]. The MRI use is mainly reserved to diagnose complicated placenta previa, such as previa-accreta and previa-percreta [37].

16.2.1 Recommendations for Management of PA (American College of Obstetricians and Gynecologists, 2018) [38]

- Standardized approach with a comprehensive multidisciplinary care team at tertiary care centers with blood bank, and intensive care unit with experienced obstetricians, urologists, interventional radiologists, obstetric anesthesiologists, critical care experts, general surgeons, and neonatologists.

- The optimal timing and number of ultrasound examinations in suspected placenta accreta spectrum are unclear. A reasonable approach is to perform ultrasound examinations at approximately 18–20, 28–30, and 32–34 weeks of gestation. This allows for the assessment of previa resolution, placental location to optimize timing of delivery, and possible bladder invasion.
- Cesarean delivery is followed immediately by cesarean hysterectomy before the onset of labor, and a window of 34 0/7–35 6/7 weeks of gestation is suggested as the preferred gestational age.
- The role of preoperative placement of catheters or balloons into pelvic arteries for potential interventional radiologic occlusion also is controversial. Iliac artery occlusion has been reported to decrease blood loss in some, but not all, case series. Because serious complications such as arterial damage, occlusion, and infection may occur, routine use is not recommended.
- Vertical skin incisions for better access and visualization are preferred. Reasonable alternatives are wide transverse incisions such as a Maylard or Cherney incision. Inspection of the uterus after peritoneal entry is obtained is highly recommended to discern the level of placental invasion and specific placental location, which allows for optimizing the approach to the uterine incision for delivery and likely hysterectomy. Whenever possible, the incision in the uterus should avoid the placenta.
- Whenever hysterectomy is necessary, a total hysterectomy is required because lower uterine segment or cervical bleeding frequently precludes a supracervical hysterectomy.
- Best ratios for blood product replacement are 1:1:1 to 1:2:4 strategy of packed red blood cells:fresh frozen plasma:platelets. The use of autologous cell-saver technology is an option, particularly now given that theoretical concerns regarding safety and risks from fetal blood and other debris have been reduced with current filtering technologies.
- Tranexamic acid 1 g intravenously within 3 h of birth and second dose may be given 0.5–23.5 h later if bleeding persists.
- Hypogastric artery ligation can be difficult and time consuming, although it can be easily performed by experienced surgeons. The use of interventional radiology to embolize the hypogastric arteries in cases of persistent or uncontrolled hemorrhage may be useful. Interventional radiology is especially helpful when there is no single source of bleeding that can be identified at surgery.
- Other methods to tackle severe and intractable pelvic hemorrhage include pelvic pressure packing and aortic compression or clamping. Pelvic packing, although

not standard management, can be highly effective for patient stabilization and product replacement when experiencing acute uncontrolled hemorrhage. Packing may be left in for 24 h (with an open abdomen and ventilatory support) to allow for optimization of clotting and hemostasis. Aortic clamping is likely best reserved for experienced surgical consultants or heroic measures given the potential risk of vascular related complications from this approach.

- Postoperative period requires extreme vigilance for complications such as postpartum hemorrhage; renal failure; liver failure; infection; unrecognized ureteral, bladder, or bowel injury; pulmonary edema; and diverse intravascular coagulation. Attention to rare possibility of Sheehan syndrome is also warranted.
- For patients with focal placental adherence, removal of the placenta by either manual extraction or surgical excision followed by repair of the resulting defect has been associated with uterine preservation. Alternatively, placental removal followed by insertion of a Bakri balloon was successful in preventing hysterectomy in 84%.
- In patients with more extensive placenta accreta spectrum, expectant management is considered an investigational approach. With expectant management, the cord is ligated near the placenta and the entire placenta is left in situ, or only the placenta that spontaneously separates is removed before uterine closure. Data are limited to case series when evaluating expectant management. The degree of success with *expectant management*, defined as leaving the placenta in situ, of placenta accreta spectrum appears to correlate with the degree of placental attachment abnormality.
- *Adjuncts to conservative and expectant management* included uterine devascularization with uterine artery balloon placement, embolization or ligation, and postdelivery methotrexate administration.
- For expectantly managed patients with persistent placental tissue with or without substantial bleeding, hysteroscopic resection of the placental remnants has been proposed as an adjunctive treatment. Given these limited data, the frequency of adverse events, and the proportion of patients who needed a repeat procedure, routine hysteroscopic resection with or without antecedent high-intensity focused ultrasonography is not recommended.
- Delayed interval hysterectomy is a derivative of an expectant approach to placenta accreta spectrum, except that future fertility is not a consideration, and minimizing blood loss and tissue damage is the primary goal. Patients with placenta percreta are optimal candidates for this procedure because they have an increased risk of blood loss and tissue damage if hysterectomy is performed at the time of cesarean. But the data is limited and it should be considered only after proper counselling and in tertiary care center.

Recommendation	Grade of Recommendation
Diagnosis of Placenta Accreta Spectrum	
Although ultrasound evaluation is important, the absence of ultrasound findings does not preclude a diagnosis of PAS; thus, clinical risk factors remain equally important as predictors of PAS by ultrasound findings.	1A Strong recommendation, high-quality evidence
It is unclear whether MRI improves diagnosis of PAS beyond that achieved with ultrasonography alone. Accordingly, MRI is not the preferred recommended modality for the initial evaluation of possible PAS.	1B Strong recommendation, moderate-quality evidence
Women with suspected PAS diagnosed in the antenatal period based on imaging or by clinical acumen should be delivered at a level III or IV center with considerable experience whenever possible to improve outcomes.	1B Strong recommendation, moderate-quality evidence
Management	
Optimal management involves a standardized approach with a comprehensive multidisciplinary care team accustomed to management of PAS.	1B Strong recommendation, moderate-quality evidence
Delivery at 34 0/7–35 6/7 weeks of gestation is suggested as the preferred gestational age for scheduled cesarean delivery or hysterectomy absent extenuating circumstances in a stable patient. Earlier delivery may be required in cases of persistent bleeding, preeclampsia, labor, rupture of membranes, fetal compromise, or developing maternal comorbidities.	1A Strong recommendation, high-quality evidence
In the setting of hemorrhage, data from other surgical disciplines support the use of a range of 1:1:1 to 1:2:4 strategy of packed red blood cells: fresh frozen plasma: platelets.	1A Strong recommendation, high-quality evidence
Conservative management or expectant management should be considered only for carefully selected cases of PAS after detailed counseling about the risks, uncertain benefits, and efficacy and should be considered investigational.	2C Weak recommendation, low-quality evidence

Key Points

1. Asherman's syndrome occurs mainly as a result of trauma to the gravid uterine cavity determining its partial or complete obliteration.
2. The development of intrauterine adhesions is associated, in approximately 90% of cases, with intrauterine curettage after pregnancy.
3. Asherman's syndrome is associated with a high risk of severe pregnancy complications such as spontaneous abortion, recurrent pregnancy loss, preterm delivery, intrauterine growth restriction, uterine rupture, and even placenta previa or accretism.
4. Hysteroscopy and office hysteroscopy represent the gold standard both for diagnosis and treatment of Asherman's syndrome.
5. The incidence of placenta accreta in patients with previous Asherman's syndrome was estimated to be 13–14%.
6. Complications of delivery including placenta previa were significantly higher in patients with a history of Asherman's syndrome compared with controls.

References

1. Asherman JG. Amenorrhoea traumatica (atretica). BJOG. 1948;55(1):23–30.
2. Wallach EE, Schenker JG, Margalioth EJ. Intrauterine adhesions: an updated appraisal. Fertil Steril. 1982;37(5):593–610.
3. March CM. Intrauterine adhesions. Obstet Gynecol Clin N Am. 1995;22(3):491–505.
4. March CM. Management of Asherman's syndrome. Reproduc BioMed Online. 2011;23(1):63–76.
5. Kjer JJ. Asherman syndrome in a Danish population. Acta Obstet Gynecol Scand. 2014;93(4):425–7.
6. Al-Inany H. Intrauterine adhesions: an update. Acta Obstet Gynecol Scand. 2001;80(11): 986–93.
7. Taskin O, Sadik S, Onoglu A, Gokdeniz R, Erturan E, Burak F, Wheeler JM. Role of endometrial suppression on the frequency of intrauterine adhesions after resectoscopic surgery. J Am Assoc Gynecol Laparoscopist. 2000;7(3):351–4.
8. Roy KK, Baruah J, Sharma JB, Kumar S, Kachawa G, Singh N. Reproductive outcome following hysteroscopic adhesiolysis in patients with infertility due to Asherman's syndrome. Arch Gynecol Obstet. 2010;281(2):355–61.
9. Yu D, Li TC, Xia E, Huang X, Liu Y, Peng X. Factors affecting reproductive outcome of hysteroscopic adhesiolysis for Asherman's syndrome. Fertil Steril. 2008;89(3):715–22.
10. Zikopoulos KA, Kolibianakis EM, Platteau P, de Munck L, Tournaye H, Devroey P, Camus M. Live delivery rates in subfertile women with Asherman's syndrome after hysteroscopic adhesiolysis using the resectoscope or the Versapoint system. Reprod BioMed Online. 2004;8(6):720–5.
11. Nitabuch R. Beiträgezur Kenntniss der menschlichen Placenta. Stämpfli'sche: Buchdruckerei; 1887.
12. Bencaiova G, Burkhardt T, Beinder E. Abnormal placental invasion experience at 1 center. J Reprod Med. 2007;52(8):709–14.
13. Bajwa SK, Singh A, Bajwa SJS. Contemporary issues in the management of abnormal placentation during pregnancy in developing nations: an Indian perspective. Int J Crit Illness Inj Sci. 2013;3(3):183.
14. Tantbirojn P, Crum CP, Parast MM. Pathophysiology of placenta creta: the role of decidua and extravillous trophoblast. Placenta. 2008;29(7):639–45.
15. Strickland S, Richards WG. Invasion of the trophoblasts. Cell. 1992;71(3):355–7.
16. O'Brien JM, Barton JR, Donaldson ES. The management of placenta percreta: conservative and operative strategies. Am J Obstet Gynecol. 1996;175(6):1632–8.
17. Kastner ES, Figueroa R, Garry D, Maulik D. Emergency peripartum hysterectomy: experience at a community teaching hospital. Obstet Gynecol. 2002;99(6):971–5.
18. Oyelese Y, Smulian JC. Placenta previa, placenta accreta, and vasa previa. Obstet Gynecol. 2006;107(4):927–41.
19. McComb PF, Wagner BL. Simplified therapy for Asherman's syndrome. Fertil Steril. 1997;68(6):1047–50.
20. Capella-Allouc S, Morsad F, Rongieres-Bertrand C, Taylor S, Fernandez H. Hysteroscopic treatment of severe Asherman's syndrome and subsequent fertility. Hum Reprod. 1999;14(5):1230–3.
21. Fernandez H, Al-Najjar F, Chauveaud-Lambling A, Frydman R, Gervaise A. Fertility after treatment of Asherman's syndrome stage 3 and 4. J Minim Invasive Gynecol. 2006;13(5):398–402.
22. Miller DA, Chollet JA, Goodwin TM. Clinical risk factors for placenta previa–placenta accreta. Am J Obstet Gynecol. 1997;177(1):210–4.
23. Wu S, Kocherginsky M, Hibbard JU. Abnormal placentation: twenty-year analysis. Am J Obstet Gynecol. 2005;192(5):1458–61.
24. D'Antonio F, Iacovella C, Bhide A. Prenatal identification of invasive placentation using ultrasound: systematic review and meta-analysis. Ultrasound Obstet Gynecol. 2013;42(5):509–17.

25. Comstock CH, Love JJ Jr, Bronsteen RA, Lee W, Vettraino IM, Huang RR, Lorenz RP. Sonographic detection of placenta accreta in the second and third trimesters of pregnancy. Am J Obstet Gynecol. 2004;190(4):1135–40.
26. Gielchinsky Y, Mankuta D, Rojansky N, Laufer N, Gielchinsky I, Ezra Y. Perinatal outcome of pregnancies complicated by placenta accreta. Obstet Gynecol. 2004;104(3):527–30.
27. Levine D, Hulka CA, Ludmir J, Li W, Edelman RR. Placenta accreta: evaluation with color Doppler US, power Doppler US, and MR imaging. Radiology. 1997;205(3):773–6.
28. McLean LA, Heilbrun ME, Eller AG, Kennedy AM, Woodward PJ. Assessing the role of magnetic resonance imaging in the management of gravid patients at risk for placenta accreta. Acad Radiol. 2011;18(9):1175–80.
29. Warshak CR, Ramos GA, Eskander R, Benirschke K, Saenz CC, Kelly TF, Resnik R. Effect of predelivery diagnosis in 99 consecutive cases of placenta accreta. Obstet Gynecol. 2010;115(1):65–9.
30. Tikkanen M, Paavonen J, Loukovaara M, Stefanovic V. Antenatal diagnosis of placenta accreta leads to reduced blood loss. Acta Obstet Gynecol Scand. 2011;90(10):1140–6.
31. Engelbrechtsen L, Langhoff-Roos J, Kjer JJ, Istre O. Placenta accreta: adherent placenta due to Asherman syndrome. Clin Case Rep. 2015;3(3):175–8.
32. Baradwan S, Baradwan A, Bashir M, Al-Jaroudi D. The birth weight in pregnant women with Asherman syndrome compared to normal intrauterine cavity: a case-control study. Medicine. 2018;97:32.
33. Feng ZC, Yang B, Shao J, Liu S. Diagnostic and therapeutic hysteroscopy for traumatic intrauterine adhesions after induced abortions: clinical analysis of 365 cases. Gynaecol Endosc. 1999;8(2):95–8.
34. Thurmond A, Mendelson E, Böhm-Vélez M, Bree R, Finberg H, Fishman EK, Goldstein S. Role of imaging in second and third trimester bleeding. American College of Radiology. ACR Appropriateness Criteria. Radiology. 2000;215:895–7.
35. Simon EG, Fouche CJ, Perrotin F. Three-dimensional transvaginal sonography in third-trimester evaluation of placenta previa. Ultrasound Obstet Gynecol. 2013;41(4):465–8.
36. Dawson WB, Dumas MD, Romano WM, Gagnon R, Gratton RJ, Mowbray RD. Translabial ultrasonography and placenta previa: does measurement of the os-placenta distance predict outcome? J Ultrasound Med. 1996;15(6):441–6.
37. Warshak CR, Eskander R, Hull AD, Scioscia AL, Mattrey RF, Benirschke K, Resnik R. Accuracy of ultrasonography and magnetic resonance imaging in the diagnosis of placenta accreta. Obstet Gynecol. 2006;108(3):573–81.
38. Placenta Accreta Spectrum. Obstetric Care Consensus No. 7. American College of Obstetricians and Gynecologists. Obstet Gynecol. 2018;132:e259–75.

GPSR Compliance

The European Union's (EU) General Product Safety Regulation (GPSR) is a set of rules that requires consumer products to be safe and our obligations to ensure this.

If you have any concerns about our products, you can contact us on ProductSafety@springernature.com

In case Publisher is established outside the EU, the EU authorized representative is:

Springer Nature Customer Service Center GmbH
Europaplatz 3
69115 Heidelberg, Germany

Batch number: 10370708

Printed by Printforce, the Netherlands